HINDSIGHT IN 2020

Surviving Advanced HPV Anal Cancer

By

Bonnie Lane (yes, me too)

Dedicated to all those who have braved this rare, often stigmatized cancer and the brutal, outdated treatment regimen of Chemo Radiation and/or APR surgery.

There must be a better way.

Copyright

Disclaimer

The reader is advised to discuss the comments on these pages with his/her personal physicians and only act upon their physicians' advice. This book is not intended as a substitute for the medical advice of a physician. The reader should regularly consult a physician in matters related to his/her health and particularly in respect to any symptoms that may require diagnosis or medical attention. The author and publisher disclaim responsibility for any adverse effects directly or indirectly resulting from the information contained in this book.

Table of Contents

Introduction

I have had this recurring dream for about as long as I can remember. I am being chased by a faceless, formless, invisible enemy. I run from it. The fear I feel is debilitating and renders my legs useless. It is gaining on me. It is right on my heels. Just before it catches me, I remember – I can fly! I know that I can, and *it* cannot. *It* has limitations. I do not. At the last second, right before it catches hold of me, I put my running into another gear and flap my arms as hard and fast as I can, and I lift off the ground. I rise up and barely make it to the top of a tree, but I am safe for now. I wake up in a cold sweat, but with a feeling of triumph.

I long felt as though I would face a catastrophe of some type at some point in my life. I also knew I would possess extraordinary skills to survive it. As a legacy, I would help others to survive. This was not a dream. This was more of a premonition. I feel very strongly that it is here now. Is it my cancer diagnosis? Will I survive it and help others with my knowledge? Perhaps. Will my enrollment in this specific clinical trial pave the way for a cure for others in the future? I hope so. Is it this Covid virus that is infecting millions? I don't know. However, it is curious that both are due to viruses – viruses that are faceless, formless, invisible enemies.

They have limitations. *We* do not.

Prologue

I write this book to entertain but mostly to provide insight into your cancer journey. Cancer does not have to be a detriment to our lives. It can be the catalyst to turn one's life around and see it from another vantage point. It's a chance to rebuild and declutter those things which are not important and to rediscover those which are. It is a chance to take the stress out of your life and replace it with gratitude and joy, a chance to give back by helping others with your newfound knowledge. The amazing healing benefits you will receive are just a bonus!

Hindsight in 2020 begins with a history of my past. As a young girl coming of age in a big city like Chicago, I had numerous encounters with men. Any one of these incidents could have given me this deadly HPV virus which caused my Anal Cancer. Some of those encounters were not of my own undertaking. The "Me Too" movement has only added to my desire to tell this story, and you will see that I hold a special place in my heart for those not empowered enough to say no or for those who have been sexually assaulted. Often with young girls, it can be both. This message runs like a thread through my life.

The book will focus on the devastating time I was first told "you have Anal Cancer," to my frantic attempts to find an alternative cure. Follow me through the brutal conventional treatment, to the metastatic return, and ultimately to my control of that cancer. All this happening within the backdrop of a devastating, worldwide viral pandemic. It details both my intense physical and emotional traumas and how I eventually started to heal both. From a layman's point of view, it touches on my opinion of a flawed medical system. Whatever happened to the original Hippocratic Oath, "First, do no harm?" And it treads ever so cautiously into my future.

Hindsight will introduce you to countless pioneers that are paving the way to new protocols to treat cancer, both conventionally and alternatively. Fellow warriors are trying a myriad of novel approaches to cure or control their diseases in an attempt to keep their immune systems intact and perhaps survive until a cure is found. Most experts say a cure for cancer is just around the corner. What does that mean? These cures include Immunotherapy, both natural and chemically derived, targeted therapies, cancer vaccines, tumor-infiltrating lymphocytes (TIL), cytokines, CAR T-cells, CRISPR-Cas 9, and the use of off-label drugs to metabolically starve our cancers et al. No more high-dose chemo and radiation, please! No more unnecessary biopsies and surgeries! Our bodies are designed to heal themselves! Our immune systems are the answer and always have been. So, let us help them do what they are designed to do.

If only I knew then what I know now!

Hopefully, this story will touch your heart, heal your spirit, and breathe new *hope* into *any* cancer diagnosis.

If you have recently been diagnosed with advanced cancer and time is of the essence, please skip over my background and start with Chapter 10. In the most urgent cases go directly to the end of the book to the section titled *Recap for those Newly Diagnosed with Anal Cancer* **or** *Tips for those Newly Diagnosed with Any Cancer.*

Part I

Gravity

Chapter 1

Foundation

My earliest memories are those of my mother. Perhaps this is because I *had* to hang on to those. They are snippets of moments that I had with her. One is of her bouncing me on her hip while she cooked. Too many of my memories, however, center around fear. On at least one occasion, she wanted my daddy to spank me. As I laid bare bottomed across his lap, he instructed me to cry while he slapped his own leg. I performed. My daddy was a kind man with a heart of gold. I recall several fights between my mother and my oldest sister Barb, who was a teenager at the time. During one episode, the bedroom door was slammed so hard the entire flat shook. I was inside the bedroom with Barb, and my mother was attempting to scold her. Mom was enraged. She threw four heavy iron stove grates at the door while Barb held it shut with a dresser and all her weight. Our door never closed properly after that incident. Spankings were commonplace, and the weapon of choice was usually a wooden spoon or my dad's belt. We used to hide the spoons inside our boots in the hall closet. Mom and Barb fought over everything; her chores, piano lessons, homework, and boys. I shared a bedroom with my oldest sister for several months while my middle sister, Marnie, fought and mercifully survived a serious childhood illness, Rheumatic Fever. As sisters, we shared a common threat, our mother. This was the dark side of my childhood, and back then, we didn't talk about it.

My dad met my mother in Germany where he was stationed in the Army during WWII. As a young soldier, he and his buddies frequented the local bakery where my mother worked. My mother, Maria, was stunning. She had a strong resemblance to a young Ingrid Bergman. Maria was the daughter of Frau Theresa and Herr Peter Eder. They were the purveyors of a bier and limonaden (soda) factory in Sauerlach (a suburb of Munich). My opa (grandpa) had died in his twenties, and my oma (grandma) was raising three children on her own (Peter Jr., Maria, and Rese). I knew little of my mother's childhood; only that which her sister, my tante (aunt) Rese, spoke of. She was said to have had extreme anger issues even as a child. I understand that she took after my opa. I was told that she once hit her older brother over the head with a chair, severely injuring him. He was too afraid of her to ever retaliate.

In my mind, I pictured a love story between my parents. I regret not asking my dad more about his life before us, or his time with my mother. What I do know is that they were married in a quaint chapel in the Alps after the war ended. He had served as an MP, charged with rounding up Russian POW's after the war. He said that he started to let most of them go when he found out what was happening to them. Some of them had already hung themselves. The Russians treated most of those prisoners as traitors to the Nazis, and either sent them to their deaths or to the Gulag, which was likely a fate worse than death. When my dad was done with his tour, he returned with his new wife to his home in Chicago. They moved in with my grandmother where Barb was born. Soon they bought a six-flat building on the corner of Diversey and Greenview in Chicago's Lakeview neighborhood (my childhood home). This was a very smart move and probably at my mother's direction. Five of the flats were rented out, and they lived in one of the two-bedroom units. Despite always desiring a boy, they had three girls; Barbara, a brunette, Marnie, a redhead, and myself, a blonde. Our names were chosen ahead of time and had to be changed when we were born. I was supposed to be Frankie and ended up Bonnie. My dad told me that my birth was difficult for my mother as I was a vaginal breech (bottom's up). This must have been quite traumatic for both of us! Barb is ten years my senior and Marnie three. As the baby, I was spared most of the punishments that were inflicted on them. Barb experienced the worst of my mother's rage.

Our family was incredibly involved in the church and school that we attended. It was the St. Bonaventure Catholic Church and School just down the street from our home. I recall my dad bringing boxes of fruit from our bountiful garden to the rectory. Our garden was lush with fruit trees and perennials back then. I can still smell the Lily of the Valley, Lilac, Rose, and the vibrant Forsythia in spring. We had apples, pears, peaches, cherries, rhubarb, and strawberries, to name a few. Perfectly trimmed hedges lined our manicured lawn with a large rosebush smack dab in the center. Our home and garden were always organized and impeccably clean. My mother was clearly the authoritarian figure in our home. My dad spent a lot of time in our garden while my mother tended to the house, cooked, and baked. She was a wonderful baker. I often fell asleep or woke up to fabulous smells coming from our kitchen.

I recall playing Ring Around the Rosie, running through a sprinkler, and soaking in a kiddie pool in the summers. We also had a painted playhouse with ruffled curtains sitting on top of a flagstone patio where I often played with my Tiny Tears Doll. I won that prized possession at my father's annual company Christmas party. My raffle ticket number was one of the first called, and I had a whole stage of gifts to pick from. There were bicycles, wagons and lots of expensive toys, but I chose the doll. You put water in her, and she cried real tears!

It seemed like my mom was overly concerned about outward appearances. My sisters told me that when company came to the house, we were treated much differently. Mom and dad had some German friends who had a son my age. We played together often while our parents socialized. I have many pictures of Reinhardt and me in our Sunday best clothing with perfectly coiffed hair, holding hands in our living room. It was as if our parents were grooming us for marriage one day.

I was born in 1959 and my mother became ill in 1964. She was diagnosed with AML, Acute Myelogenous Leukemia (a cancer of the blood). There was no cure for it back then, and she only lasted months after the diagnosis, leaving me motherless at the early age of six. My most vivid memories are of her death and seeing my dad cry. That really affected me. I also recall the funeral and my oma coming over all the way from Germany. That was no easy trip in 1965. The nuns from my school came as well, and marching behind them was my entire first-grade class!

My sister, Barb, will be forever traumatized by my mother's death. As an adult, she confided in me that she often prayed at night for God to take my mother when she was younger. The guilt of that after mom died has been a weight that she has carried throughout her life.

For the three of us, we clung to our father like there was no tomorrow.

"No one ever told me that grief felt so like fear."

C.S. Lewis

Chapter 2

Trials

After my mom passed, nothing was ever the same. Some things were better, others worse. My oma insisted that we come to Germany for the entire summer when I was just eight years old. Just the three of us girls went. It was such an experience to travel to a foreign country at such a young age. I had cousins a bit older than me to play with, and we stayed with my grandmother in the brick, two-unit farmhouse next to their Bier and Limonaden factory.[x]

My aunt and uncle lived downstairs from my oma with their son Bader (Peter), who was 14 at that time. There was an above-ground pool in the yard where we had loads of fun. I loved to watch the bottles in the factory as they went through the assembly process, and to accompany my uncle on deliveries to meet all the quirky town's people. We would often stop for homemade treats made by locals along the way. It was a fascinating adventure.

We played with our cousins and had many fabulous meals, and even got to drink beer with our meals. I got sick one time and hugged the toilet all night. Beer is like water to Germans. We went hiking in the Alps, mushroom picking in the forest, and rode our bikes around town. My aunt had matching Dirndls sewn for us girls. Those are the colorful, cute Alpine peasant dresses with the high tight bodice and full skirt with an apron.

Unfortunately, I recall being sexually molested by my cousin Peter in the woodshed (of all places.) Before I knew it, he had pulled out his penis and put his hand down my panties. I ran out of that shed, ashamed and frightened. I so looked up to that boy and had such fun with him at the pool. It was a one-time thing, and I told no one, but I will never forget the incident.

We stayed for the entire summer. My dad and aunties laughed at me because I forgot how to speak English for a while when I came home. It was a crude form of German that, as a child, I picked up in just a few short months.

After our trip to Germany, my dad's older sister, Irene, came to help him. Auntie "I" was so different than my mother. She had no children of her own and lost her husband not long after they were married to Parkinson's disease. She had a kind heart like my dad, but like my mother, she also butted heads with Barb. About a year after my mom's death, Barb, still just a teenager, got pregnant and left home with a boyfriend.

My dad worked nights at a factory as a machinist. The arrangement was that after school, my dad would drop us off at our busha's (grandmother in Polish) house, and my auntie Irene would bring us home when she got off work. Busha owned a four-flat building with a tavern on the first floor, and since my grandfather had already passed, she lived in the back apartment with her oldest daughter, my auntie Jennie.

My auntie "I" lived in one of the upstairs apartments. My auntie Jennie and busha ran the bar. We spent about two to three hours there on weekdays. What memories! The bar, the patrons, the spittoons, the old coin-operated bowling game with the puck and sawdust, the jukebox with the songs I will never forget *Roll out the Barrel, Mack the Knife, Beer Barrel Polka*, buying penny candy from the general store down the street, and getting hot dogs from the "putt-putt" vendor. We often drank fountain coke and ate bagged chips at the bar tables. Our family parties were held in the backroom where we helped our busha cook. This was the Polish side of my family.

My grandparents came over from Poland in the twenties during prohibition. They first owned a general store and sold moonshine out back. They would tell us stories of how the authorities once came to do a routine check, and they piled all the liquor onto the bed and sprayed perfume on it. The kids were told to get under the covers with it. When liquor sales were finally legal, they opened the tavern and closed the store. 'Jean's Place' was named for my aunt Jennie. My first paid job was stocking those coolers for a dollar an hour! There were shelves for beer and even a shelf for aunt Jennie's homemade pickles. Back then, they fed the patrons. Anytime busha and her daughters cooked, everyone would eat! It was always a feast. We often ate pierogis, sauerkraut, and golumpka (cabbage rolls). Once a year, right before Easter, we made massive amounts of Polish sausage. It was an event. All the aunts and uncles came over and participated. I loved to hold the casings as the grinding machine filled them.

I always felt as though I was my auntie's "favorite." She had a soft spot for any wounded bird or underdog, and I certainly fit that bill with two older sisters often picking on me. I recall them making me do their chores, cutting my hair while I slept, stealing my treats, and tickling me until I cried. *How I hated that!* Unlike my mom, my auntie "I" never worried about how I was dressed or what my hair looked like as long as I was clean and well-fed. When I was eight, she taught me to play Poker and Gin Rummy for a halfpenny a point. We played cards for hours together on many occasions.

My aunt watched us for a few years until we got older, and she could no longer handle us. With Barb out of the house, my sister Marnie, now 14, was put in charge of me after school. Marnie was bossy with me initially, but I was a tough kid and stopped listening to her early on. From about the age of 11, I spent quite a few hours unsupervised each day.

I had a life-altering event happen the year I turned 11. I was walking home from school one spring day without a care in the world. I never had a fear of strangers until after that day. I was as close to home as I could get when a man grabbed me from behind and forced me into my own gangway. A gangway is a long narrow sidewalk that connects two properties. That name is interesting, and I wonder where it came from. Did gangs assemble there? I can't imagine that. Our gangway was especially long and dark as our two-story brick building was tall, and we sided to another large brick building with a car wash.

The man showed me a big hunting-style knife. He put it back in his pocket and held it to my stomach through his jacket lining to conceal the weapon. He unzipped his pants and told me that he would not hurt me as long as I did what he asked and did not cry out. Paralyzed by fear, I did what he asked. He forced me to put my mouth on his penis. The only other time I had seen a penis was when my cousin molested me, and I had tried my best to forget that! I had no idea why he made me do this, but I knew it was very wrong. I wished that my daddy was there to help me, but no one was home. I wonder if this man knew that. Next, he put his hand into my panties. I felt so helpless and afraid. He rubbed me in my private area. I don't remember if he ejaculated into my mouth or on the ground. I think it was a combination of both, but I will never forget the smell. To this day, I wretch at that odor.

It was probably all over very quickly, but it did not seem that way to me. I went home, locked all the doors, took a long bath, and cried until my sister came home. I was frightened and embarrassed about what had happened but did my best to act normal around my family. That night I had a dream that shook me. A faceless, formless enemy was chasing me. I ran from it. I was terrified by it. The fear I felt was debilitating and made my legs useless. It was gaining on me. I could feel it right on my heels. Then I remembered, I can fly, and it cannot. I suddenly put my running into another gear and flapped my arms as hard and fast as I could. I lifted off the ground and made it to the top of a tree. I was safe - for now. I woke up shaking and covered in sweat.

Some people say that you can't have the same dream twice, but that's not true. I had that dream many times after that. Where I landed sometimes changed, but most of the details remained the same. I could fly, and my invisible enemy could not. I felt like it was a man chasing me, but when I looked back, there was never anyone in sight. I saw the man that assaulted me one more time on my way home from school. He was walking toward me. This time, he was with another man, and I was with a friend. Our eyes met briefly. I was crippled with fear. The look he gave me was, as best as I can describe, playful, as if we had some type of secret bond. I wanted to run and fly like in my dreams, but I stayed grounded and never looked back. The most interesting part is that I never mentioned a thing to my sister, dad, auntie, or anyone for that matter until I was 15 and opened up to my freshman counselor. She was young and approachable and formed a safe environment for me.

Eventually, I would tell friends, but only after things had happened to them. I had a friend who was raped and tied to railroad tracks near her home. She freed herself and managed to make it home to her parents. Her dad acted like it never happened, and they never talked about it as if he was ashamed. *How awful*, I thought. My story was nothing compared to hers, but her story convinced me not to come out to my family. I never told my dad, but I often wonder how he would have reacted. I can only guess that he would have blamed himself for not being home. I loved my daddy, and it didn't make sense to tell him after all those years had passed. It does not surprise me when women don't open up about rape or molestation for years. I believe them. They don't want to talk about it for fear of a variety of repercussions. Why would anyone lie about a thing like that? I totally believe Christine Blasey Ford[i] when she says that Brett Kavanaugh raped her, and I understand why she had not said a thing all these years until, of course, she felt she had a strong reason to do so. She was so credible in my eyes! And I feel that I am more of an expert than most!

Actually, I was quite a tomboy back then. My sister and I befriended a family of seven Italian boys down the street from us who we grew up with as great friends. While my sister had more of a love interest with the older boy, Mark, I was often the only girl playing baseball, football, and drinking beer with the others. They had a fort above their garage where we used to drink beer, smoke pot, and listen to music. They were good boys from a solid family, and I developed a big crush on Mike. We often made out but never took it any further. I remember my aunt caught us making out one time by our side gate, and she chased him with a broom down the street!

"It's hard to trust when all you have from the past is evidence why you shouldn't."

Dpsayings

Chapter 3

Identity

When I was in the fifth grade, some of my classmates and I formed a group that would fill small bottles with liquor and mixers and meet in the bathrooms between classes at school to drink them. We made Harvey Wallbangers, Whiskey Sours, Highballs, and other such drinks. We pretended we were grown up and drinking fancy cocktails. Our parents had no idea that we were stealing their booze. Unfortunately, one day I left my pencil case in my desk while changing classes, and a boy in my class found it and innocently turned it in to the teacher. The teacher opened it, and I got busted! In it was a small vanilla bottle filled with Seagram's 7. I was the first girl in the history of my catholic grade school to ever get suspended. The other girls could not believe that I never ratted on them, but I simply took the punishment and became extremely popular with the boys after that! My dad was disappointed, but I sensed that he also thought it was just a slight bit humorous.

In middle school, I had a blast. I had two good friends at school, but my bestie was Janelle, who lived down the block from me. Janelle did not go to my catholic school. She went to the nearby public school, but somehow, I was still the instigator of trouble. We were inseparable. Since there was no parental authority at my house, my sister and I became quite popular with our friends. We would hit my dad's liquor and replace it with water. We would smoke his cigars too. Yuk! I will never forget the first time I tried one, and like an idiot, inhaled it. I got so sick! I despise the smell of cigars now, but I like the taste of Cognac!

We had our boyfriends in middle school and kissed them and pretended to be in love. We played 'Spin the Bottle' at parties and went to the beach in the summer scantily clad in our bikini tops and cutoff jean shorts. Our bikes were our mode of transportation. It was a short bike ride from where we lived to Lake Michigan where sandy beaches and many friends awaited us. This was a weekend ritual during the Chicago summers. Someone always brought a big boom box, and we blasted our rock music, drank beer, and smoked joints wrapped in psychedelic-colored papers. Janelle and I would curl our hair, put on makeup, and hang out with much older kids. I almost lost my virginity at 14 with a guy in my basement, but my dad caught us. I know now that this boy or man should not have taken advantage of me even though I was a willing participant. He was 18, and I was still a child according to the law. He could have been charged with statutory rape, but this did not deter him. My dad really went through a lot trying to raise three girls without a wife! I, alone, put him through hell.

I ended up going to an all-girl catholic high school, Notre Dame for Girls, that required a 40-minute bus ride to and from home every day. I ended up becoming friends with the "druggies." We were adventurous and thought drugs made us look cool. We wanted to look older than we were. I have never regretted attending a catholic school. I made some good friends and have held onto those friendships throughout adulthood. My best friend Janelle moved away when I was 15 and remains the last best friend I had in my life.

At 15, I met a boy near my home named Randy, who I would lose my virginity to. He introduced me to heavier drugs. He let me drive his car, and I got into an accident before I even had a license to drive. We did manage to switch seats quick enough for him to take the blame, though. After his Kentucky-bred mother started talking marriage at such a young age, I broke it off with Randy after only about a year. No way I was getting hitched that young. I heard later that he got into injecting heroin, and I truly hope that was not because of me.

My high school friends and I went to concerts, hung out with boys, and partied at the forest preserve. The movie 'Dazed and Confused'[ii] perfectly depicted those years of my life. I worked weekends in retail and saved for my first car. It was a '72 Oldsmobile Delta 88 convertible. It was like a boat and fit a slew of girls in it. What fun we had driving around in that car with the top down.

A section of our large basement was decorated with our old furniture, a floral rug, black lights, and posters. We had a turntable where we played our favorite rock albums. We had a lot of great parties in that basement, but my 16th birthday was my favorite! I invited a combination of high school and neighborhood friends. We sang, danced, and drank all night. Whenever I hear a Bob Dylan song, it reminds me of that night when we were all singing at the top of our lungs, *Everybody Must Get Stoned*.

We experimented with many different types of drugs in my high school years. We were completely and utterly fearless. I had a few different boyfriends back then. Boys often coerced me to do things I wasn't comfortable with. Why I let them, I don't know. It was, after all, a time when women were marching in the streets for equality. I liked to think of myself as a tough and independent girl, but I did not speak up when push came to shove. Was it because I was under the influence of drugs and alcohol? Was I afraid of looking inexperienced? Probably a little bit of both. You would think that after being molested when I was younger, I would have learned to say stop. Unfortunately, that was not the case.

I ended up meeting Paul at a bar when I was 17. I had a fake ID, of course. He was four years older than me and so handsome. We fell in love quickly and spent every minute together. I was incredibly lucky that I did not get pregnant. We did not use condoms regularly or think about consequences to our behaviors. I'm not sure what I would have done if I had gotten pregnant in high school.

I had always planned to go away to college, but that never happened as I didn't want to leave Paul. Most of my high school friends went to Southern Illinois University, and to this day, I regret not going. It would have been a chance for me to gain some more independence. For a few years, I took some classes at Northeastern and Wright Junior College, but that was not comparable. I got good grades, but I had no plan for any specific career.

I always found it more comfortable to be around boys than girls. I never saw myself this way, but my girlfriends always called me the "pretty one," and while it was a compliment, it also came with a stigma. How I hated being lumped into the "dumb blonde" stereotype. I had a lot of high school friends, but no one was super close. I was envious of others who had a tight bond with a friend or sister. On some occasions when I thought I was building a friendship with someone, my feelings would get hurt by something they said or did, especially if I felt "left out." With my sisters, we always vied for my dad's attention, and we fought a lot. I was happy when my sister Marnie got married, and it was just my dad and me at home. My dad quit his job at the factory when his plant moved to Rockford. He just didn't want to travel that far from home. I don't think my dad knew what he was going to do for a job. My dad's brothers were all Chicago police officers. He may have felt a bit jealous of that, as he passed the physical but did not pass the psychological test. As a young driver on the streets of Chicago, it suited me well that my uncles and a cousin were cops. I got out of all my tickets! All I had to do was show my last name. Two of them were sergeants!

My dad and I went to the racetrack a lot after he quit his job. I learned how to read a program at an early age, and my dad would make small bets for me. I would yell at the finish line for my horses to nose out their competitors. It was great fun. One day at the track, my dad ended up befriending an Italian guy who was most definitely mob-related, but we all loved him. My dad confided in him about losing his wife to cancer, and Jimmy, in time, became my dad's best friend. Jimmie employed my dad as a bookie which was the income that supported us for years. He never had to deal with the ugly side of the business. He just took sports bets over the phone, collected losses, and paid out when they won.

I remember one time he got tipped off that the feds were coming, and he wasn't home, so he called me and told me to take certain papers and flush them down the toilet. I did what I was told, but some of the papers did not flush! The cops suspected me of doing just what I did and then found more papers and money. They waited for my dad to come home, and he went to jail. But, with his contact, he was out within hours. Jimmy assured me of that.

I would take care of my dad and the house as best I could until I got married and left home. My dad did the best job that he could with three girls and no wife. He somewhat neglected our building and backyard, but we always had hot meals and a roof over our heads. We could have used a bit more supervision, but we never lacked for love. Had my mother been alive, we would have had plenty of supervision. We would have had music lessons, college degrees, and would have been living in the suburbs long before then!

The disco scene was in full force at that time, and one of my high school friends and I used to frequent the clubs on Rush Street on the weekends. It was crazy fun. We drank, we danced, and we met men with money. Without naming names, I once met a member of the Bears football team and took a ride with him in his fancy sports car. We started kissing, and before I knew it, he unzipped his pants and pushed my head down into his lap, hard. He forced me to give him the worst blow job ever. I spat it out on him when he was done. I hated him for that. It was as though he expected it – stupid me for getting in the car with him in the first place.

I met another young man at a bar that we frequented. He was the most popular and best-looking young man at the club. I had seen Tony many times before and admired his dancing. I was so taken aback when he asked me, of all people, to dance with him. He taught me some of his moves, and we danced together all night. When the club closed, we kissed outside and went to his car to get out of the cold. After making out for just a brief time, he forced himself on me. I tried to open the car door and leave, but I was overpowered. Feeling absolutely humiliated for trusting him, I went home with torn panties and shaking with anger. Repeatedly, I made the same stupid mistakes.

In some ways, I experienced more before I was 21 than most women experience in a lifetime.

"It was not your fault, even if you were drunk, even if you were wearing a low-cut mini-dress, even if you were out walking alone at night, even if you were on a date with the rapist and kind of liked him but didn't want to have sex with him."

Joanna Conners

Chapter 4

Emotions

After five years of dating, Paul Cantelli and I were married in October of 1980. I had the whole shebang – including a crazy weekend with my friends at the Kentucky Derby for a bachelorette party. I can't get into the details of that weekend because what happens at the derby stays at the derby! We also had a huge shower thrown by my mother-in-law-to-be. She was a special person and so very generous. I miss her very much.

It was highly unusual, but it snowed on the day of our wedding. It was a beautiful church and ceremony. I wore an antique white gown, and my bridesmaids were dressed in a rich maroon color. My two sisters attended along with my best friend Janelle who came in from Minnesota to be my maid of honor, and my high school friends Carol and Leah. It was a lovely ceremony. Paul was half Italian, but it was the dominant half, so we had a BIG Italian wedding. We had 450 people at our reception! That's huge! I remember not knowing many of them. I guess they were friends of our parents.

The event was held at the Aqua Bella Banquet Hall on Harlem Avenue in Chicago. Jimmy and all his friends came, and with Paul's family, it was a large, boisterous Italian wedding. We raked in a lot of cash. Italians, for some reason, try to outdo one another with wedding gifts! It was enough to buy a car and then some. We were fortunate enough to start off in a brand-new condominium in the north suburbs of Chicago.

Paul worked for his uncles in a remodeling business installing aluminum siding and gutters, and I encouraged him to go out on his own. So, we started a new business called Windy City Construction. He worked from home, and I worked for the Riviera Hotel while helping Paul with his books and paperwork. The Riviera Hotel was a posh, Las Vegas hotel back in the day, and they had a Chicago office that booked group travel, junkets, and collected debts from its VIPs. I worked for an Italian man who was also "connected." Another girl and I attended all the VIP parties, and we often got confused with the hired women. There were many celebrities at those parties. I remember meeting Bill Cosby at one event, and it did not surprise me when I heard he was accused of sexual assault. He was quite flirty with the hired young ladies. We socialized with the men and let them order bottles of Dom Perignon for us. The laugh was on them when our boss came over and told them that we were his "secretaries."

We won a couple of "all-expense paid" trips to Las Vegas by booking the most hotel rooms of any remote office. We flew first class, got picked up in a limo, could eat at any restaurant, and order room service anytime. This was the decade of cocaine. My bosses' friends had plenty to share. I never got hooked on coke or any drugs, for that matter. I liked to do just a little to fit in, but I was most definitely a lightweight. I saw many of my friends and my husband get addicted.

At 24, my high school friend Fran and I decided to open a business together. We called it "Gourmet Express." It was a lunch delivery and corporate catering business. The lunch delivery business was a novel idea at that time as no one was really doing it. At least not in the burbs. I borrowed money from my dad, and we filled the kitchen with used equipment. We hired drivers and cooks, and off we went. Fran was a great cook, and I handled the paperwork and took orders. We shared most of the other duties. But, unfortunately for the business, I got pregnant shortly after we opened and had a baby in the mix.

Paul and I did not try to get pregnant. I simply forgot to take my pill. Michelle was our "happy accident." I always felt as though I had great "willpower." I smoked cigarettes, drank, and took drugs when I wanted to party. But, at age 25, I quit all of it when I got pregnant.

I had a healthy and normal pregnancy except for my last month when I developed an awful rash that started on my stomach and spread to my entire body. I went to the dermatologist, and he told me that I was allergic to my baby and that it would go away as soon as I gave birth. He said that he could give me something to help the rash to go away but that it could be bad for the baby. Without hesitation, I decided to grin and bear it. I took several oatmeal baths a day and slathered on the calamine lotion afterward. Paul and I went to Lamaze classes, and I decided to try and have my baby naturally without pain meds. During labor, I thought I was dying. My back hurt so much that I threw up several times. I fought hard and did my breathing exercises, but my labor was nearing 20 hours, and I finally took an extremely low dose of something to ease my pain. I did not even consider an epidural since there was a risk of respiratory distress to my baby.

After Michelle was born, I decided to breastfeed her, even though it would be difficult with the new business. I believed strongly in the immunity benefits of breastfeeding. Michelle Marie was born on August 8, 1985, and completely and utterly stole our hearts! We loved and cared for that baby like no other. Just like her birth, she was not an easy baby, as she was colicky and cried endlessly every night right before bedtime. Perhaps she felt the stress I was under dealing with the problems at Gourmet Express and the guilt of bringing her to a sitter's house five days a week. I know that's what working parents did and like the Helen Reddy song said, "I am strong, I am invincible, I can do anything, I am woman!" But I still had a challenging time with it.

I returned to work as soon as possible, and even brought Michelle with me for a few months. It was very rough having a business partner during this time. I was also experiencing some post-partum depression. Fran and I butted heads over many catering jobs and I'm sure she did not love the fact that I had a baby, husband, and home that stole my time away from the business. She often put in many more hours than I did. We ended up selling after five years, and it was quite a blow to our friendship.

Shortly after Michelle was born, I realized that a third-floor walk-up condo was not ideal for a family, so we bought our first home. We bought a lovely old four-bedroom, two-bath house in a nearby suburb of Chicago. We made it our own. I had some experience growing up in a six-flat building, but our Wolf Road house was where we learned how to do rehab work, and we loved it. The before and after made me want to do more projects.

After we sold the lunch delivery and catering business for a decent profit, I used the money to begin my next career in residential real estate. It made the most sense since I had a child and could make my own hours. I liked it and was good at it. I knew by a fairly early age that I liked working for myself.

At 28, I got pregnant again. Not planned, of course. Anthony was born on July 24, 1988. He was the first boy in our family. For years we did everything with and for our children. I may not have been the best parent, but I loved my children, and they knew it. My parenting skills included little structure. They sometimes went to work with me, stayed up late at night, and often slept in our bed. I fed them healthy meals and insisted that they try everything. I wanted them to grow up strong and independent, so I did not shelter them from experiences. As the first boy in a family full of girls, Tony never lacked confidence and was spirited from the get-go.

Our kids played some sports and took music lessons, but they were never committed so nothing lasted. We had a lot of parties with family and friends at our home, including a big, annual Fourth of July party with a pig roast, volleyball, music, and fireworks. We had to invite several neighbors so that they did not call the police on us. Our family vacations often involved camping and the outdoors. We took the kids fishing, rafting, biking, swimming, and hiking. These were incredibly happy days for all of us.

My auntie Irene was so much like a mother to me and a grandmother to my children. I was lucky to have her in my life. She was a smoker her whole life, and it finally caught up with her. She developed congestive heart failure and ended up in the hospital a few times with breathing difficulties. We finally convinced her to give up smoking. Not long after she did, she had a stroke. I guess when you smoke that long and then quit, it can be a shock to your blood vessels. She never recovered from that stroke, and I felt guilty for making her stop smoking.

She had a written will (however crude it was) and often verbalized her wish not to be put on any life support. She was in a catholic hospital at the time, and I was in charge of making decisions for her. It was challenging for me when I had to take her from the hospital and put her in another facility to die. She would not have wanted a feeding tube, so we did not let the catholic hospital put one in, and because of this, they would not treat her any longer. I spoke to her doctor at the new facility, and he agreed that she was not likely to recover. She could not talk, walk, or feed herself. She did not recognize us any longer, or at least I don't think she did. I visited her daily and did my best to feed her, but her organs would soon shut down. They say that people do not feel hunger in this state, but my only thought was that she needed food. I had a tough time with that. I was too young to be making those kinds of decisions. In the end, my dad and I knew in our hearts that she would not want to live this way. I was with her at her bedside when she passed. This has left a scar on my heart that will stay forever. As far as I was concerned, she was the only mother I ever really knew.

As our kids got older, our marriage started to experience more difficulties. We were in our thirties now and seldom spent time alone together; our time was always with the kids. This was probably a mistake. We grew apart in many ways. We had purchased another home as an investment. One of our renters was a single woman. It seemed that Paul was spending a great deal of time doing repairs at the house. Well, it just happened that he was getting a little something in exchange for the rent money. Of course, he denied it, but he was never a good liar. I got a new tenant, and we never heard from her again. It was odd, but I was not as upset as I should have been.

I needed a change and spotted a new adventure. It seemed like gambling was always a big part of my life, and I developed a strong attraction to it. I enjoyed the environment and the personalities of gamblers. Casinos were starting to open in the Chicagoland area but only allowed on the waterways as floating casinos. The stories of dealers making big money in tips were appealing to me, and I decided I wanted to become one. Applications were being taken for a new casino in Elgin, IL. The Grand Victoria Riverboat, owned by Caesars Entertainment, would be the next big gambling venue to hit the area. I applied, was trained, and opened the new boat in 1994 as a blackjack dealer.

The first couple of years were so much fun. It's what I needed to put some energy back into my life. Of course, this took me away from home for more hours than my real estate career. My kids did not seem to mind as they had their friends and activities. Their dad was in charge on the days that I worked. My schedule consisted of four ten-hour days, and I was off for three. It seemed like there was always a party or meet-up at a bar after work, especially on the weekends. I did not feel guilty about being away from home since the kids were already asleep. It was, after all, wind down after being on our feet for hours on end and dealing with drunks and pathetic losers. Oh, the stories I could tell about those patrons. Not everybody knew how to keep gambling in check, and the greed aspect ran through from the corporate owners on down. One time, when I was on a break, a fellow dealer was in the restroom crying and washing her foot off in the sink. She told me when she was what we called "dumping" money on her table. Everyone was winning and having an exciting time, and suddenly, she felt a warm wet sensation on her foot and leg. She soon realized that a man at her table had urinated on the floor and hit her leg. *OMG, WTF! They can't even leave the table to go pee!*

I usually worked the high-stakes blackjack table, but I also, after a certain time, became proficient at dealing Baccarat, Roulette, and Caribbean Stud Poker. One time, while dealing blackjack, I gave a customer 80 thousand in just a couple of hours. He proceeded to give it all back plus another 20 thousand before leaving and cussing me out because he tipped me so much while he was winning. He wanted the tips back. Of course, that did not happen. More craziness happened like you wouldn't believe. Messages often came over the paging system when patrons left pets in their cars or children in the adjacent movie theatre unattended. Once, we had a man have a heart attack and die at my table. The other patrons wanted the table to stay open, so they only closed off half the table. *Really?*

Anyway, the job was a total blast for a couple of years, and I made great money. I have been told that I was quite a looker in my late thirties. I worked off all the weight I had put on with my children. Since I had a job in customer service, I always maintained perfect hair, nails, and makeup. Men were attracted to me, and I liked it.

This one time, I did have a plan. The plan was to have an affair and feel better about having been cheated on myself. I had a crush on a handsome co-worker, and a regular customer was also in the running. One night, my friend wanted to meet a customer for a drink after work. She asked me to come along. He brought a friend, so I ended up sitting with him. We talked for hours, and because it was his birthday, I kissed him at the end of the night. He started to come to the boat quite often after that. On one occasion, he asked me what number to play on the roulette wheel, and I said, "put your money on nine." As a kid, I always liked Randy Hundley, the catcher for the Cubs, and his number was nine. He put down a twenty-five-dollar chip on the nine, and I rolled one! The odds are thirty-five to one! It was exciting. He told me that he wanted to tip me after work so that I did not have to split with all the other dealers. I met him after work, and we kissed again. I knew that night that my affair would be with Ben.

Our affair lasted way too long. Things did not go quite as I had planned. I fell in love or lust or maybe both. Ben was very charming and quite a bit older than me. That's why I initially thought he was the safest choice. He was recently divorced and so different than anyone I had ever been attracted to in the past. He was an athlete and enjoyed gambling as I did. He was generous and especially thoughtful in bed, often paying much more attention to my satisfaction than his own. I was not used to that. Our meetings were quite clandestine, and often this only enhanced the excitement. The excitement turned into fear and guilt. I wanted to break it off several times, but I couldn't. I became quite attached to him. My home and marriage were suffering, and I had to make a choice. I was forced to lie about everything I did, and I couldn't keep it up much longer. I decided to tell Paul that I was in love with another man. In retrospect, I acted impulsively. I acted with my heart and not with my head. I thought that Ben would be more on board with my decision. I know that he did not want us to break up, but he also did not want to be responsible for breaking up my marriage. Ben thought I was insane for telling Paul. He knew what it was like after having been through this himself with his ex-wife. Of course, in that situation, she got caught and then confessed.

My decision to come out about my affair did not go well at all. Duh! Paul's mom and my dad got involved. For the sake of the family, Paul and I agreed to go for counseling. The advice from family was, of course, for me to break it off. The advice from the counselor was for Paul to quit smoking pot (which he was very much addicted to) and for us to continue counseling. He tried to quit smoking and began tackling some of his other demons. I cut ties with Ben. Paul did *not* want the divorce, and we tried to make the marriage work. It was increasingly evident that it would not succeed. He began to follow me, and I was frightened that he would hurt me. He punched the pillow next to my head so hard one night, and I knew it was meant for my face. He later admitted that he had purchased a gun. One day while cleaning the garage, I found notes that he had made as part of his therapy regarding mistakes he needed to own up to. I read them, screaming aloud as I discovered so many secrets that I now wish I had never seen. It was mind-blowing.

A man I trusted for so many years had deceived me for most of my married life. I wanted a divorce immediately. I talked to his mom and tried to tell her about my reasons without divulging Paul's secrets. She did not need to know those things about her son. Deep down, she understood because she was also divorced. Paul's father was a drinker and a cheater, and she had remarried years ago. She forgave me. Many people did not. Because of my affair, many of our friends and relatives blamed me for the divorce. Of course, I blamed myself too. It was the kids that made everything so hard. I was so full of guilt for what I was putting my children through. I cannot stress this more. I was so full of guilt for what I was about to put my children through.

"Above all, be the heroine of your life, not the victim."

Nora Ephron

Chapter 5

Trust

My divorce was finalized in 1998 when my kids were just 10 and 13. I wish I had waited longer for my kids' sake, as it was difficult for both of them, especially for Tony. He was a lot like me, very emotional. Michelle had a close set of friends, and I think she faired a lot better, but who knows what damage was done. She did not open up to me about it. As for myself, I always felt the guilt, and I was not prepared for the loneliness. I had not even considered how much of an outcast I would become. Because Paul came from such a large, tight-knit family, we did a lot together. Birthdays were always celebrated and holidays plus weekends at the cabin in the summer. It was something that his mom insisted on. She was the glue that kept the family together. They were an interesting bunch. They had their own imperfections for sure, but I was now the enemy. In the old-world Italian family, a woman rarely cheated on her husband, let alone divorce him.

There were many nights that I cried myself to sleep, wondering why I did what I did. My kids wanted to be with their cousins, aunts, uncles, and grandparents. I was no longer invited to those parties, and I could not ask my kids to stay with me. I had Ben now, but at what cost? I had plenty of doubts that bordered on complete regret.

They say that divorce is often as bad on one's psyche as the death of a close relative. For me, I found this to be true. It left scars on me that took years to fade. I thought Ben could have helped me heal quicker, but he did not understand what I needed from him. He pushed back, thinking I was trying to smother him. We went to counseling to try to work through our issues, but we never did. I wanted to trust him, but first, I expected him to prove his love for me. It ended up taking years for me to feel that I made the right decision. If there was ever a time in my life where stress overwhelmed my immune system, this was it. I felt that I was looking for "unconditional love" from Ben, which he was incapable of giving. I had a few anxiety attacks, which were petrifying, losing control like that.

We did our best to get through this period. We took the kids to counseling and even bought them a puppy. Our beagle pup, Xena, ended up helping me to get through this tough time. She had a way of knowing when I was sad, and I got my "unconditional love" from her.

I took a trip to Jamaica with just myself and the kids. I wanted them to know that none of this had anything to do with them or our family unit. I wanted them to know that now they would have two homes and not one less ounce of love. Paul moved into our rental house, and I stayed in the main house with the kids. The agreement was for them to stay with me during the week and with their dad on weekends.

It was at this time that my son started to get into real trouble. Of course, all the therapists warned Paul and me about staying consistent and in agreement in our parenting. This did not happen. Tony would play us against each other, and when he did not get what he wanted from me, he would complain to his father, and when we punished him, his father would take Tony's side. His dad filed papers for custody, and instead of letting it go to court, I gave in and ended up letting our son live with his dad for a whole summer at just 16. It was a horrible idea. Paul wanted to be his friend, and I understood this at a certain level, but Tony needed discipline and structure. He got into more trouble with drugs, alcohol, and authority. Of course, I felt the guilt of this. He got his first DUI at just 16 when he lived with Paul. I helped him to pay his fines and made him do the required counseling and community service. When he returned to live with me, he stole cash from Ben's pockets and my retail business. He pawned my jewelry, some of which was left to me by my aunt. This was devastating to me that he could stoop this low. I am sure now that not all of this was due to the divorce.

Tony was always a precocious kid. From an incredibly early age, he could lie like a pro. He had a kind heart and was extremely generous, but he lacked honesty. He lied because he was impulsive and wanted things. He did not think through the consequences. I'm sure Tony had plenty of fun in high school, but he also had an addiction propensity, just like his father. During this time, I did not spend enough time with Tony, not that he wanted to spend time with me. I simply did not put enough effort into getting him the help that he needed. I see my mistakes now but at the time, I was caught up in my relationship issues with Ben.

Ben had been living in a bedroom in his mother's house when I met him and spending a great deal of money on sports betting and vast amounts of time golfing. Obviously, he loved me, but he was also quite happy with his bachelor's lifestyle. I talked him into buying a home with the money he had left from his divorce. Financially, it was a great decision. At my suggestion and with my expertise and help, we rehabbed the home and sold it for a 40% profit in just about a year. He then moved in with me but was still not ready to fully commit to our relationship, and by that, I mean marriage. It was mainly because of his daughter and ex-wife and partly because of my insecurities and my son's behavior toward him.

It was also around this time that I was told that I had some abnormal cells when getting the results of a routine pap smear. I needed to come in for further testing. After that testing, it was determined that I had some pre-cancerous cells on my cervix and needed an office procedure called a LEEP (loop electrosurgical excision procedure). My gynecologist would freeze the area and slice off a small portion to remove those cells. It was not that uncommon, and it would take just an hour, and then I would need a pap smear every three months for the next two years to make sure we got it all. I recall now that she told me after the test that it could be from a virus called HPV and to eat my green vegetables. I didn't know much about HPV back then, and I was too busy with my life to worry about something that was now supposedly gone.

It was around this time that my good friend, Jodi, was diagnosed with Breast Cancer. We were all devastated to hear that she would need surgery and chemotherapy. She was living alone at the time and had no one to take her to appointments and surgery. I took her to her surgery and helped her wash her hair after. Yet now, I wish I had done much more for her. I can't imagine how it must have been to be alone for all her follow-up treatments and scans.

I quit my job at the casino and bought a business. It was time, as the environment was not healthy for me. Most people thought the new business was too risky, including Ben, but I was confident in my abilities. What I lacked in knowledge and experience, I more than made up for with hard work and common sense. I had already helped Paul run a successful construction business, and I operated Gourmet Express with Fran, so I knew I could do this. I had a special knack for managing money, and I soon realized that I also was quite tuned in to what was trending with the public. These qualities suited me well throughout my life. With my dad's financial help, I bought a deli in an office building where I provided corporate catering along with breakfast and lunch to the occupants of the building. I also facilitated the vending and ATM services. My daughter and her friends worked there in the summers, and it kept me busy and gave me some much-needed confidence. It felt good to hear how much the customers loved my specials and sandwich creations. That deli was a great little moneymaker. I easily tripled the business that the previous owner was doing, and my dad became a regular customer. He loved to sit and watch the customers and tell them that I was his daughter. I tried to pay him back, but he wouldn't accept the money.

At 41, after two years of divorced life, I married Ben. It was not the proposal nor the ceremony that I had envisioned, but it was lovely. We were married on a beach in Puerto Vallarta with our children. Ben's parents joined us. To my great disappointment, my dad would not make the trip. He did not like to travel that much, and when he made up his mind about something, there was no fighting him on it. It was a far cry from my first wedding, but this was a different time. It was a second marriage for both of us. Our families were small, and since my divorce, many of my old friends were now divided. I regret not having a bigger celebration of our union together.

"Peace begins in your heart, grows in your mind, manifests through your will, and spreads through your action. "

Anna Pereira

Chapter 6

Tribulations

Life had changed dramatically for me. I had Ben, and we did love each other, but was love enough? I was often both sad and lonely and longed for the feeling of belonging to a close family unit. The holidays were especially hard on me. I often wondered if I had made the right decision divorcing Paul, but deep down knew I could not be with Paul again. In retrospect, I probably should have learned how to live alone and not depend on any man for my self-worth. I went from my dad to Paul and now straight to Ben. I was no "Helen Reddy!" I expected Ben to make me feel whole again. He did not. He could not.

Sex with Ben was great. I have read that women are not in their prime until their late thirties. I believe that to be true in my case. I need to mention that Ben had a growth that would occasionally appear on his upper buttocks/lower back area. He said that he could feel when it was coming on. We joked about it being some type of herpes, but I did not worry about catching it since it was on his back. He said that he got it from a tanning bed before he met me. I knew that he already had it when I met him, but I never really believed the tanning bed story. We tried to avoid it. I should have been more careful. Well, I did catch it. I used to blame him when I got the bumps. I felt a tingling sensation in my nerves right before the breakout. They itched at first and then hurt a little. Mine would show up right where I sat on the lower part of my buttocks. I think I may have caught it when I sat on his back and gave him a back rub in bed. I realized now that I should have taken this more seriously. The bumps came and went, normally lasting a few days and then dried up. I would seem to go months without an outbreak, and then when I was feeling under the weather, they would pop up. They came about when my immune system was low. I had heard about others with herpes that just dealt with it, and so would I.

I had some challenges with employees at my deli. I caught one of them stealing from me, and another was found to be soliciting young men at the mortgage company in our building to have sex with his wife while he watched. It became a scandal in our office building. I had one devoted and reliable employee, and when she started to have problems showing up for work, I had had enough. I sold the deli, banked my profits, and took a few months off to contemplate my next career. During this time, I also decided that Ben and I needed a home of our own. My home was filled with too many memories of my old life with Paul and the kids.

We sold my home in Des Plaines for a substantial profit and turned around and put all that money down on a newer home with a big lot in Schaumburg. Michelle, now away at college, came back home for summers. Tony, once again, found it hard to adjust and did not like leaving the one and only home he had known, not to mention his friends. He was not happy with the move. He got a second DUI and blamed it on me for moving.

I figured out quickly that if I wanted to spend time with Ben, I had to learn to golf, and he was more than willing to be my teacher. I learned to love the sport. I started to play in lady's leagues and met many new and needed friends. Ben was still my best friend. He was a good man. He was never a drinker, and I came to realize that he was also not a cheater. He was simply addicted to golf, and I learned to live with that. I gave up a lot of the "old me" to be with Ben.

We spent a great deal of time golfing and sometimes gambling. Our friends were golfers as well. When we traveled, it always centered around golfing and gambling. As for the gambling, we knew how to leave when we were up, which most gamblers did not do. We also knew when to take our losses. You can't keep chasing.

Xena loved the new house. We were on a half-acre, and she had a great big yard to run around in. We also took her for two walks every day through the neighborhood. She was getting older for sure, and we hated to see her develop Cushing's disease. The vet wanted to put her on a medication that caused severe side effects, and I wanted to look for an alternative. Many experts agree that Cushing's in dogs can be caused by processed dog food. It does not contain the nutrients they need. I took this diagnosis as my personal journey into curing her of this disease. I started to research everything I could about Cushing's and tried switching her to a raw diet but found out that it was too late in her life to switch her diet that drastically. I decided to start her on a supplement designed specifically for Cushing's and start making homemade food. I used my own oils and supplements to add to it. I made it with brown rice, fresh vegetables, salmon oil, and a quality powdered multivitamin. She thrived on that diet and then developed some type of heart issue.

The vet again wanted to put her on some strong meds, and I said no. I researched again and started to treat her with a naturopathic blend of cayenne pepper, curcumin, and other supplements. She did well on them. A few years later, she developed a tumor on her side, and it grew quickly to about the size of a golf ball. I took her in to the vet, and we had it biopsied. They told me that it was cancer. Xena was 16 now, and there was no way that she was going under the knife. It was also an expensive surgery, plus the tests and medications. It just made no sense to put her through all of that at her age. She also still had a decent quality of life. She loved her walks despite her slow down. She absolutely loved to eat, and she still played on occasion. I started to research natural cancer therapies. It seems that humans and beagles are not all that different when it comes to cancer.

Cancer is cancer. It is when your cells start to grow uncontrollably. I must admit that I was a bit over my head in this research, but I did stumble upon an inexpensive protocol by a German woman named Johanna Budwig[iii]. It seems overly simplistic, but Dr. Budwig was an expert in fats at the cellular level. Joanna Budwig was a biochemist and pharmacist who held doctorate degrees in physics and chemistry. She developed a diet that she believed was useful in the treatment of cancer. She was one of the first to realize that the low oxygen environment in cells only encouraged the proliferation of cancer cells, so she tried to change the environment of those cells to an oxygen-rich environment. She was nominated seven times for the Nobel Prize in medicine and dedicated her life to studying the healing effects of Omega 3 oils.

I knew that all pets and humans were deficient in Omega 3's and that we had an overabundance of Omega 6. Because our food underwent so much processing, it no longer supplied us with certain necessary nutrients. I started to make Xena the Budwig Protocol every day. It is a mixture of organic cottage cheese and fresh flax oil, to which I added freshly ground flax seeds. I mixed those ingredients with an immersion blender and gave it to her on a spoon. She loved it. After about three months of this, she developed a fistula in her tumor, and putrid yellow pus began to seep from it. I would simply wipe it away. Slowly the tumor disappeared. It was amazing.

After selling my business, I took three months off before looking for another income. It's not that we needed the money, it's just that I wanted to retain my independence. I had used a

Business Broker to sell my business. It sold quickly, and the broker took a whopping 10%! I knew that this was something that I could do, so I investigated what I needed to become a broker for business sales. This varied from state to state, and luckily for me, there were no huge requirements in Illinois except to pay for a license and renew it each year. I interviewed with Sunbelt Business Brokers and got the job. I would need to attend some training from them, and I would be paid by commission only. I would start with a 50/50 split with Sunbelt, where in exchange, I would be provided with the training, a desk, computer, conference room, and a shared administrative assistant. I was going to be the only woman in the office other than the admin.

My first year was challenging to say the least. It was difficult getting business owners to trust you. It was frustrating working with buyers as they had absolutely no loyalty to working with you, and there was no one source for listings. As a result, unlike residential real estate, most business brokers advertised, listed, and sold their own listings. In my second year, I developed the confidence to list, market and sell a few small businesses. I started out selling restaurants, later shifting my focus to include liquor stores, salons, and spas. It could often take months or even years to make a sale, but when I did, it was very lucrative. I was comfortable being around men, and most of them respected me after I started to sell more substantial businesses such as pharmacies and manufacturing companies. After a time, I got to where I could talk to almost any business owner and earn their respect with my knowledge of their financials. Business owners love to talk about the value of their businesses.

After the market crashed in 2008, the banks got tight with money, making it difficult for buyers to obtain financing. It got a lot more cutthroat in our office, and leads were often doled out by our boss. I started to feel like I rarely got a good one. They all seemed to be going to the top two or three selling brokers so that they would not leave. I resented this. I had a few issues at work with my boss. One sale cost me 30,000 dollars in commission. One of my listings was sold to a buyer I brought in, but I did not have a signed confidentiality agreement. It was a technicality that he would absolutely not have imposed on certain other brokers, and everyone in the office knew it. I was livid. I could have sued for discrimination, but I was not sure if I could win. I let it go, but for me, it was never the same after that.

Michelle had graduated from college and was working and sharing an apartment with friends in the city. Tony tried a year at college, but he got caught drinking a few times on campus and could not keep up on his grades. He also got a third DUI which cost us more in legal fees. This time he paid for it with his college fund left to him by my aunt when she passed. He was 19 now and an adult. His drinking was spiraling out of control. I was done with bailing him out. He did not complete his required community service and would this time be facing arrest. I did not pay his bail, and he ended up spending two weeks in Cook County Jail! I cried when they took him away in handcuffs, but I could no longer be his enabler. I explained to him why I did this, and I hoped he understood. I think this may have been quite a wake-up call for him.

I recall one time that he called me and told me that I needed to phone Jamica at a certain phone number and tell her that Darius would meet her at a specific location and time. I said, "No, Tony, I'm not going to do that." And he said, "Mom, you don't understand. I NEED you to do this." I understood that Darius was standing right next to him, and Tony was afraid, so I made the call for Darius.

Tony eventually moved out when he was 19 to an apartment in Chicago to access public transportation to travel to work. Obviously, his license was now revoked. He did not hold any job for exceptionally long, but he somehow stayed above water by working odd jobs. My children were both out of the house now.

At that time, Ben's dad was in and out of hospitals with one thing or another. He was not a healthy man. He ended up with liver failure and passed away. Ben took this awfully hard, and for the first time, I saw him cry. He was not one to look for comfort from me; instead, he withdrew into himself and pushed me away when I tried to console him. Finally, I decided it was best to let him handle his grief in his manner.

Soon after that, his mom got ill. It often goes that way with couples. One goes, and the stress and heartache that the other experiences can manifest into dire health issues. Ben's mom had macular degeneration and dementia, so it was difficult for her when she needed a knee replacement. She was having a harder time seeing, and she could no longer drive. We often had to bring groceries and take her to appointments. Mom ended up passing about two years after dad.

It was around this time that a good friend of mine was diagnosed with Lung Cancer. We were close with Cindi and Josh. They were our favorite golf buddies. I was shocked when I found out that Cindi had Lung Cancer. She was truly fortunate to have caught it as early as she did. Most Lung Cancers are not found until they are at stage 3 or worse. Hers was stage 2, and there were two small tumors; one about the size of a dime and the other a quarter. Since I had healed Xena's cancer a few months back, it seemed reasonable to look up the effects of the Budwig Protocol on Lung Cancer. What I saw online was incredibly positive, and what could it hurt? I sent her everything I could find on the benefits of Omega 3 oils. Of course, she would follow her doctor's recommendations, but she also did what she could to help herself. I was proud of her. She quit smoking and started on the Budwig program. She also had a holistic healer friend who sent her a combination of essential oils that she had to rub on her chest every night. She did it all. She had surgery to remove two-thirds of her lung, and we visited her in the hospital the day after her surgery. She was quite agitated that day, and who can blame her. Not only did she have major surgery, but she also had not had a cigarette or drink for days. She was in full withdrawal. She spent most of our visit pleading for more pain relief. It was a long and hard recovery for her, but she recovered. She was fortunate that she did not need to do any chemo or radiation. She later developed neuropathy, and her lung function was never the same, but she was alive and had a rather excellent quality of life.

Ben was now approaching retirement age, the kids were out of the house, and my job at Sunbelt was annoying me more and more, so we investigated moving again. This time we wanted to downsize, and since we loved golf, we started to look at golf properties. Our dream was to live on a golf course somewhere. We looked a bit in the suburbs of Chicago, but anything decent was unaffordable. The taxes were especially high in Illinois, and so we contemplated moving out of state. The only thing stopping me was my dad. He was getting older, and I did not want to leave him alone. I got him to promise to come live with us as soon as he felt he could not live alone any longer. I felt that my kids no longer needed me. Lastly, I was starting to develop a chronic bronchial issue that was worse in very cold temperatures. My doctor called it "cold-induced asthma." That was enough to make me want to leave Illinois.

We searched the map for affordable homes on quality private and semi-private golf courses. We took several trips to

Florida, California, Alabama, Utah, and Arizona. We needed it to be somewhere warm with low taxes and reasonable golf fees. Ben's daughter was in Nevada now and married with two children. With Ben's advancing age, it made sense for us to be closer to her and the grandchildren, so we settled on Prescott, AZ.

"Regret for the things we did can be tempered by time; it is regret for the things we did not do that is inconsolable."

Sydney J. Harris

Chapter 7

Inertia

It took us about six months to sell our home in Schaumburg. We were still feeling the effects of 9-11 and the 2008 market drop and ended up selling our home for a loss. There was nothing we could do about it. The days of big gains in real estate were over. We were lucky that we could sell at all in this climate. Our new home, on the other hand, was a great buy. I knew that it would be. Homes directly on the course were selling very quickly in that area. We purchased our home sight unseen. Of course, we came out for a final inspection, and we could have bailed at that time, but we were happy with our decision and delighted with the golf course. The home was only three years old and on the ninth hole of a fantastic golf course in a lovely, planned community in Prescott, AZ.

Prescott is about 90 miles northwest of Phoenix, in what is known as the high desert. It is much cooler here than in Phoenix, but still, there are plenty of days of sunshine. The town is full of "old west" history. Back in the day, Prescott was the capital of Arizona. It was home to many famous outlaws. You learn early on that the locals pronounce it "Preskitt." The taxes on our new home were ridiculously low compared to what we paid in Cook County. We could afford to pay cash for our new home and lower our monthly debt substantially.

Working, while Ben golfed every day was not something that appealed to me, and since the cost of living in Prescott is so low, I decided to work the few leads that I had brought with me and then quit altogether. If we needed money, I could always revisit my decision. Things seemed to work out well financially. We didn't need much to live on. So, I retired at the early age of 55. We had the perfect life from the outside looking in, especially to my friends in Illinois who were still looking at another ten years of employment.

A few months into our new life in Prescott, we had to put Xena down. It was time. She was 18. I had kept her alive and healthy for nearly two decades. I never imagined she would make the move, but she did. She didn't like the desert. I think she missed the cool grass of the Midwest on her paws. She could never get used to walking on hard, hot rocks. We often took her to the golf course at night to feel more at home. She loved that. I took her death especially hard. I love animals. Ben always joked that I loved Xena more than him. I always had cats as a child. She was my first dog. As previously mentioned, we originally got her for the kids during our divorce, and of course, I ended up spending the most time with her. I took her for walks and fed her, and she slept with me at night. I developed a special bond with her. She knew when I was sad and would lay by me and comfort me, and in turn, I took care of her when she got ill and was aging.

It was difficult for me to put my good friend down, but I would not let her suffer. I always said that her favorite things were to eat, play, and go for walks with us, and if she ever lost two out of three of those things, I would do the necessary thing. She no longer wanted to play or to be picked up. She still enjoyed her walks; however slow they were. Finally, after a lifetime of loving all food which is standard with any beagle, she started to turn away from it. I knew that I had to do the inevitable. One night she threw up her dinner, and there was blood in her vomit. My first thought was that her cancer was back. I woke up Ben and said it's time, and we took her to the emergency pet clinic in the middle of the night. As we waited to see the vet, we took her outside, and she perked up a little, which made it that much more difficult. Ben wanted to take her home, but I said no. I knew it was time. Ben could not come into the room, but I could not let her die alone. I owed her that.

I stroked her velvety soft beagle ears while they injected the medications. The ukulele version of *Somewhere Over the Rainbow*[iv] by Israel "IZ" Kamakawiwoʻole was playing in the pet emergency room when she passed, and to this day, I cannot hear that song without bawling. The lyrics combine words from *Somewhere Over the Rainbow* and *What a Wonderful World*. I encourage you to listen if you have never heard him sing it. After we put her down, I found a music box playing that song and put her collar, tags, and favorite toy inside. I believe that one day I will be with Xena again and my auntie Irene too. But for now, I know that they are together, and that comforts me.

Our golf friends soon became our lives. Our children were out of state, and although we saw them a few times a year, we spent most of our special days with friends. Ben played with the men, and I played with the ladies, except for our couples' group on Sundays. After a time, those became our closest friends. I thought our mixed group would be friends forever. Whenever I made a friend in the past, it was usually for life. Instead, the group disbanded after about two years. I am still not sure why. One of the men cheated on his live-in partner, and judgments were formed when she took him back. I also heard through our grapevine that some thought me stuck up and standoffish.

I took this hard for some reason, and I felt rejected for a time. Rejection for me was always quite painful. I don't know why I was so sensitive in this regard. All I wanted was to feel like I belonged. Was I stuck up? I didn't think so. If anything, I was shy and may have compensated for those feelings by acting cool and nonchalant. It's what I knew best. I didn't like being judged. I was strongly judged by Paul's family when we were divorced. I hoped that I never hurt anyone in this way, but I probably had. We all have a past that has shaped us, and we cannot know what it is to walk in another person's shoes.

Some friends remained constant, and others came in and out of our lives. I once saw a t-shirt that I will never forget that read; *A friend helps you move. A true friend helps you move bodies.* There was a stick figure drawing of two people moving a parcel across the ground. Awful, yes, but it made its point. I would soon find out the greatest attributes of true friendship.

I missed Xena something awful, and when we returned home from golf each day, our house seemed so quiet. There is nothing better than to have a pet greet you at the door. Xena was my best friend with fur, which left an empty space in my home and heart. Ben had heard about a fellow member looking to get rid of a puppy he had purchased for his special- needs daughter. The puppy was not the lapdog that they had hoped for. It would often jump up and bite her. It would steal her socks and bras and run off with them. They were planning to put an ad on Craigslist and just give it away. I told Ben that if I saw the puppy, I would want it. That's how I am with animals. I cannot bear to see them suffer. Whenever the ads come on TV for the animal charities, I must change the channel. I cannot look at the dogs chained up outside in deplorable conditions and their sad faces looking through cage bars. I want to save them all. I had a feeling that this puppy was in the wrong home. Who in their right mind, would just give a puppy away on Craigslist after having them for several months? Haven't they formed a bond with that puppy? Ben wasn't sure that he was ready for a dog, but we finally agreed to see it.

When we arrived, the dog was let out of his kennel and into the backyard. We sat out on the patio and tried to get the dog to come to us. His name was Nicoli, and he was a purebred miniature schnauzer. Nicoli was so cute. He was about 12 pounds and already full-sized. He was a standard salt and pepper color and they had him trimmed up in a typical schnauzer cut with the pronounced eyebrows and long beard. I did not particularly care for his haircut. It seemed a bit harsh. The dog proceeded to do circles around the entire perimeter of the yard. He ran so fast that we could not even get a close look at him. He found a newspaper and started tearing it up and eating it. The owner's wife tried to get it from him, and then he threw up what he had swallowed. She finally got a hold of him and put him back in his kennel. We talked about him for a little while, and she said that they keep him in the kennel at night and during the day when they golf. I thought to myself, oh my goodness, that's excessive. I know that the husband and special-needs daughter golf almost every day. She said that the dog was jumping a lot and showed me a vinegar spray bottle that they used to keep him from jumping. That was enough for me.

I asked, "What would happen if, after a time," but she stopped me dead in my sentence.

She said, "Oh no. If you take him, he's yours. There is no giving him back!"

Wow, I thought to myself. This woman is heartless. I was going to ask, "What if her daughter changes her mind after a time and wants the dog back?" My mind was made up though, so the words never left my mouth. We were taking this puppy home with us. Nicoli was microchipped and was up to date on all vaccines. The owner threw in the kennel, food, blanket, and dreaded spray bottle. We packed him up and never looked back. I knew what this dog needed. When I got him home, I looked into his eyes and told him that his life was about to change dramatically. His eyes were dark and wild, and he didn't seem to understand at this point, but he would. In time, he would understand just how lucky he was.

We renamed him, Pita. This was an acronym for Pain in The Ass. I must admit that's what he was. We had a little spitfire on our hands; that much was certain. We put the kennel in the garage and never used it again. I used the vinegar to clean my windows. I started by taking him for two walks a day. I guarantee he was not walked very often, if at all. He had so much energy he needed to expel. When I walked him, we often stopped to talk, and he seemed to be listening to me. I kept trying to look into his eyes to see if that hard, crazy look would change. It took time, but eventually, it did change. Pita started to calm down and develop a strong bond with me. He got super protective of me, however. Every time we passed a stranger or another dog, he reacted like a complete mad dog. He barked and pulled on his leash. Eventually, I had to keep him away from strangers. Even at home, he barked at the neighbors, and any time the doorbell would ring. He got extremely aggressive with strangers. I attempted to train him, but how could I show him the love he lacked and be stern with him simultaneously? At home with just Ben and myself, he was perfect. He slept with us and laid on the couch with us, and most times, he had to be on my lap. Interesting that the previous owners gave him away because he was not a lap dog. All he needed was love and exercise.

About six months after we got Pita, I talked Ben into getting another dog. I did not want to leave Pita alone all day when we golfed. It seemed unfair to do that. Pita needed a friend. We took Pita with us to an adoption event at a Petco in Phoenix. We saw a few younger dogs in a gated area that were shown that day. We spotted a white terrier mix that looked like it was shy. It was a girl, and her name was Delilah. Delilah had a bent ear and a brown spot right over her left eye. She also had a big spot on her side and tail. Her skin was a delicate pink under her white fur. She was precious. We have always liked the band Plain White T's, and our favorite song is *Hey There Delilah.* It was an omen.

We started to play with her, and she seemed sweet. We brought Pita to her, and they got along well. This surprised us because Pita was normally so aggressive. We told the people in charge that we were interested in adopting Delilah.

"We have another family coming later today to adopt her with an appointment already," they replied.

We must have looked disappointed because they further added, "You can wait a couple of hours and if the family doesn't come, proceed with adopting her."

We stayed for another hour, and the people finally said that we could just have her. They could tell by watching us for the last couple of hours that we were good people. They told us that she was currently living in a household with several other big dogs, so she was extremely fearful. I said that she would get plenty of walks on the trails in Prescott, and they said, "Good luck with that!" Her foster parent had a challenging time walking her. I figured that probably most of this was because they were walking those big dogs at the same time.

We signed some papers, paid a small fee, and took Delilah home with us. She seemed very timid in the car and did not seem to enjoy the ride at all. When we got her back to the house, she was better but still very timid. I was told by the woman who housed her that a volunteer had picked her up in front of a grocery store. Some young boys were trying to sell her. The boys said that they found her near a highway on garbage day. It was such a sad story, and I wondered what happened to her siblings if there were any? She was now about eight weeks old and just 15 pounds. We shortened her name to Deedee. They said she was part Jack Russell Terrier for sure and would grow to about 20 pounds. That was perfect. We did not want a big dog. Pita got very jealous, so we had to pay more attention to him until he calmed down and realized that we were not replacing him. He finally learned to accept Deedee, and she started to become increasingly attached to us. She loved the cool weather, and I could not imagine her living in the valley where the heat reached into the 100's. Her coat grew thick and her legs long. The spots on her became much more pronounced. She looked as if she could be part Dalmatian. She grew to a whopping 35 pounds!

"His ears were often the first thing to catch my tears."

Elizabeth Barrett Browning

Chapter 8

Flux

In 2015, after a routine blood test, Ben was diagnosed with probable Prostate Cancer. His PSA (protein-specific antigen) levels were off the chart. I was extremely concerned for him and us. I googled everything I could on Prostate Cancer and tried to get Ben to start eating healthy. I found out and explained to him that it was a slow-growing cancer, and he could take some time making decisions. He had to go for more tests and a biopsy. These tests were quite painful and evasive. They had to go through his rectum with a special tool that would punch sections of holes into various areas within his prostate to obtain samples. It was determined that his cancer was entirely within his prostaté and did not show up anywhere else. This was good news and quite a relief. Our primary care physician, Dr. Singh, said that if it were him, he would see no-one but Dr. Emory at the Mayo Clinic in Phoenix, so that's where we headed.

After further tests, it was determined that his entire prostate gland (about the size of a walnut) was full of cancer. His doctors felt confident that they could get it all, and he would live a full life. He was given two choices, and it was a difficult decision. His choices were surgery or radiation. With radiation to his entire prostate, he would experience a slow decline (months or even years) in his ability to achieve an erection, and the cancer would most likely be completely eradicated. The radiation oncologist was certain that this was Ben's best choice. The other option was surgery, where he could be assured that they would get all the cancer (because they would be opening him up and they could see it), but there was a slim chance he would experience a sudden loss in his ability to achieve an erection. That would only happen if the surgeon felt it was necessary to remove the nerves outside of the margins of the gland itself. It would all depend on what the doctor saw when he opened Ben up. He felt confident that this would not be the case. The robotic surgery was coined as "nerve-sparing."

Dr. Emory said that even if he had to go wider with his margins, Ben's ability to achieve erections would get better in time and that, if necessary, there were pills and injections that he could turn to for help. Dr. Emory said that he would help Ben if that turned out to be the case. The surgeon was sure that this was Ben's best option. Ben had a little bond with Dr. Emory as he knew of his son, who played professional football. Ben loves sports of all kinds. They would often chat about his recent games. Together we decided on the surgery. I wanted this to be his decision, but I may have weighed in more than I should have. I just wanted him to get all the cancer, and if it were me, I would choose surgery over radiation any day.

Before we called to schedule the surgery, I talked Ben into seeing a naturopath[v]. I wanted him to look into every option. I found a doctor in Prescott who was an integrative physician. This means that he practices both conventional and naturopathic medicines. I also purchased and read a book called *Cancer, A Second Opinion* by Dr. Josef Issels. Issels was one of the first and most famous integrative oncologists. He believed in treating cancer as a whole-body disease and felt strongly that current conventional treatments were sorely lacking because they did not share this belief. I thought this type of doctor could be the best choice for Ben, but he was not enthusiastic at all about this consult. He worried about being put on a strict diet.

Dr. Zander wore Birkenstock sandals and khaki shorts, and his desk was piled with papers. He seemed like an old hippie to me, but I didn't mind that. We found out that he, too, had Prostate Cancer. I thought this was great. Not for Dr. Zander, of course, but for Ben to have someone with first-hand knowledge of what he was going through. Dr. Zander told us that this was one of the slowest growing cancers and that we had time to make decisions. He never went against the advice from Mayo, but instead suggested that we also control any possible spread by adopting an alternative protocol to go along with the conventional advice. Dr. Zander controlled his own Prostate Cancer by alternative medicine alone and checking his blood counts often to ensure it was not growing. He asked Ben about his diet and was aghast at the staples on Ben's side of the pantry. I told him that I could not get him to eat anything healthy and that I had given up years ago trying. We ate together but not the same things. We each cooked our individual meals or went out and ordered what we wanted.

It was difficult, of course, to find a restaurant that we both enjoyed. Most times, we picked up food to go and had to visit two separate restaurants. For example, Ben would get In and Out Burger, and I would go across the way and get Wildflower. His idea of a vegetable was grilled corn on the cob in season or raw carrot sticks as a snack. The meat that Ben ate was usually beef or pork. It was rarely chicken and never fish, except for deep-fried cod on occasion. He often ate frozen pizzas and take-out food (mostly hamburgers). He loved anything deep-fried and his favorite go-to meal was boxed macaroni and cheese. His normal breakfast was frosted flakes or bacon and eggs. He drank soda, chocolate milk, or orange juice. He was addicted to soda (mostly Coke). I often remarked that he had the palate of a five-year-old. Dr. Zander said that he would have to change his diet for sure. The first thing being, he would have to eliminate the sugary drinks and processed foods.

Ben did not say a word. Dr. Zander sent a list of supplements for Ben to start taking. It was all the same things that Dr. Zander was taking himself. This seemed like an easy thing to do, at least for a year or two, to make sure he got himself on the right track. He also wanted Ben to get some lab work done. I explained when we went to see him that Ben had a history of extremely high triglycerides. This was no surprise considering his diet. Dr. Zander was concerned. He asked that we get a set of labs ordered through our primary care physician. This seemed odd to me, but we did it.

I filled the order at the naturopathic pharmacy and ordered a few items online since they were less expensive. I set up a schedule for when Ben was to take them. I began cooking meals that I thought he might eat and set out his pills for him each morning. A few items were tinctures, and Ben did not like to taste anything bitter, so I had to disguise them in a chocolate banana smoothie. I made him this smoothie every morning, which he drank most of. It became increasingly difficult to get him to adhere. He would close his nose and swallow and treat me like I was the enemy for forcing him to take it. I also made him the Budwig cottage cheese and flax oil mixture; he ate it a few times but gagged while doing so.

We went to see Dr. Singh again and told him about the protocol that Dr. Zander had him on and the labs he wanted us to obtain. Dr. Singh asked Ben to consider another source. Then he backtracked his comment and said that there was no harm in his protocol. He agreed with the diet changes and expressed equal concern about the high triglycerides. However, he did not agree with many of the labs Dr. Zander wanted. This was enough for Ben to want to stop the entire protocol. We argued about this, and in the end, I gave up. It was not worth me nagging him about it. He told me straight out that he would rather die than change his diet and take those awful tasting smoothies every day. He wanted to enjoy what time he had left. I tried to tell him that his cancer was not a death sentence, but he did not see it that way. I had spent over 800 dollars and much time and effort only to have Ben refuse to take the supplements after just a couple of weeks.

We scheduled the surgery for the first week in February. It was robotic surgery, and Dr. Emory was top-notch in this field. I was curious about the surgery and found out that you could view one on YouTube. I thought that Ben would want to watch with me, but he refused. There was no way that he wanted to see that video. I watched it and found it amazing! The surgeon remotely sat at a computer with his head inserted into a tight viewing lens and worked with his own hands somehow while the patient lay on a table near him, and a large robot did the actual slicing and dicing. The robot had three arms that did the cutting and one that sucked up the blood. A few nurses kept an eye on the patient and robot, but the surgeon did not even touch the patient!

The surgery went very well, and I was by Ben's side through all the appointments and recovery. The hard part came after he healed and tried to resume some type of normal life. His golf game suffered, and he had to deal with a blow to his ego when his handicap went up, but his sex life was even more devastating. There were things that Ben was never warned about. Ejaculation was super weird. It was no longer semen. It was like watery liquid spraying out. I had no idea, and Ben was embarrassed. I told him we would figure this out together, but he withdrew more and more, not wanting to take the pills (which didn't work that well and gave him headaches) or deal with the weird ejaculation.

We talked about calling the doctor for further advice, but Ben was not interested. I downloaded several articles about different therapies for men, and there were plenty out there. He had zero desire to pursue them. I was also now in full post-menopause and experiencing dryness and pain, which is treatable but requires hormone pills or creams to be put on in advance. It was all getting to be more of a chore than it was worth. I tried to push it a few times, but Ben was not on board. He was angry and embarrassed and didn't want to talk about it. I can't imagine what it is like for a man to lose this function. Since then, he has often said that if he knew this would be the outcome, he would have done nothing at all!

With Ben's cancer and the sudden decline in our sex life, one would think that our relationship would suffer, but it actually had the reverse effect. We became closer and formed a more trusting love. He opened up to me in a way that he had never done before. I was truly open to any type of therapy or abstinence if necessary. I was leaving it completely up to him. I remember the doctor saying that erections would be most difficult right after surgery and would improve as time passed. I was holding out hope that this would happen for us.

We once again buried ourselves in our golf games and our dogs. This was our life with a sprinkling of family and travel. We would play golf five or six times a week and take the dogs for two walks a day. We watched a lot of TV and dined out often, either alone or with friends. We traveled in the winter to warmer climates. Carli, Sean, and the grandchildren visited us a couple of times a year, once in the summer and again at Christmas. My children came to visit here and there, and I also traveled to see them. Again, we had what looked like a perfect life.

We especially loved the grandchildren's visits during the Fourth of July when the town celebrated with a Rodeo and Parade. The kids ran the Boot Race downtown, and being the little athletes that they are, came home with plenty of trophies. My friend and neighbor, Hannah, came up with an idea to form a Kazoo and Lawn Chair Group and enter the parade. I was "all in" for this adventure! We formed a group of nine ladies and bought those oversized t-shirts that made you look like you were extremely well-endowed and dressed in cut-off daisy dukes with a gun holster. We all had matching cowboy hats, shoes, and red, white, and blue glitter accessories. We learned to play the kazoos in harmony and synchronize our flapping, vintage, webbed lawn chairs, and dance steps to the music. It required weeks of practice as we were mostly in our late fifties, sixties, and seventies. Our repertoires consisted of *Yankee Doodle Dandy, The Theme Song from Bonanza, The Hokie Poky, God Bless Ameri*ca, and more. We entered as the "Prescott Ladies Kazoo and Lawn-Chair Auxiliary" and got our spot in the parade lineup. We decorated two golf carts, and the grandkids rode along with their sparkly red, white, and blue attire. They oversaw handing out mini-kazoos to the children along the parade route. It was a sweltering day, and we were nervous at first, but soon settled into a fun day. As a complete surprise, we discovered just how popular we were. Each year a plaque is awarded to the best new entry, and we won it! How rewarding for all the arduous work we put into it. The judges and the crowd liked our spunk and enjoyed our routines, especially when we stopped, opened our chairs, plopped down into them and fanned ourselves, for what we called a "hot-flash time-out!". We were featured in the local paper as well.

"People will forget what you said, people will forget what you did, but people will never forget how you made them feel."

Maya Angelou

Chapter 9

Reactions

I visited my daughter in Chicago a couple of times a year. I would usually stay with my dad in his condominium. When I visited him in 2016, his dementia was getting worse. He picked me up at the train station, and his driving was sketchy at best. We sailed through two red lights, and when I brought this to his attention, he simply sloughed it off. When he parked his car in his condominium garage, I noticed a dent in the car next to him. I asked him about it, and he denied that it came from him. It looked obvious to me. He was 92 now, and my sister and I knew we had to take the car away soon. We knew that this would be a huge blow for him, as he was very independent. He lost his wife well over 50 years ago and has not answered to anyone since. One of my dad's favorite things was going to the off-track betting parlor in the old neighborhood. Even though he now lived in a condo on the far west side of the city and couldn't find his way to the grocery store anymore, his car and brain had a permanent GPS for the "Mud Bug."

When Illinois allowed gaming in casinos on waterways, they also approved off-track betting parlors for racetrack betting. It was popular with a certain subset of the community. This was my dad's happy place. He would use his handicap placard to park for free and then use his charm with the girl at the door to avoid paying the dollar entrance fee. He would bring 50 dollars with him, and it would last him all day. There's no way he would spend all that money. He was too frugal for that. Some of the money was for gambling, but some was for lending to his friends when times got tough for them. It was an interesting group. There was a roofer, a cabbie, a couple of retired guys, and of course, the millionaire. My dad liked to call him that. Everyone hung around him when he came in because he bought drinks for all or a few plates of chicken strips. It was customary to buy a plate or two of chicken tenders for the group if you were doing well on any given day. They all had their regular chairs, too (I sat in the wrong chair one time and learned that lesson).

On that same visit, I heard my dad call the middle eastern cabbie "Bin Losen" (a play on Bin Laden). I was so embarrassed, but the guy didn't care at all. I guess because it came from a 92-year-old and because everyone liked my dad. It was just his form of humor. The millionaire especially liked my dad and used to let him run bets or collect wins for him. My dad would go up to the counter and place his bets and often be told to keep the change or take a portion of a win. My dad never took the money. He just liked to brag to the other guys that he had been offered. He was happy with a couple of chicken strips and a beer.

My dad was very frugal with his money. Probably because he grew up during the depression. It annoyed him so much to see how the price of groceries went up. When we shopped for him, we could never show him the receipt. He would ask, "How much did you pay for these apples?" We would have to lie. When he went to the store, he would buy extraordinarily little for himself. It was sad. He just refused to pay those prices. He had money in the bank, but he would not spend it. Instead, he lived on a very meager pension and his social security.

We took the car away soon after my visit, and the plan was for him to come live with me in Prescott. He knew deep down that he could no longer drive and that we were doing this for his own good, but at the same time, his dementia was getting worse, and at times he just could not think straight. He would sit at the edge of his bed and just stare at the television remote. My sister had to come so many times and reset the television because he would have it so messed up. I would get so worried when I would call him, and he didn't answer the phone. His hearing was also poor. I used to call the other tenants in the building to go and check on him. One time when he did not answer his phone for a day and a half, I called the neighbor, and she banged on his door early in the morning and got no response. I then called the fire department, and they broke the door down just to find him sleeping in his recliner with the TV on full blast.

In the months before our 2016 presidential election, I started to become interested in politics. I know that many of you reading this book may not share my views and I hope this will not cause you to lose interest in my story.

While I respected the views of most conservatives, I felt strongly about this particular Republican candidate. In my opinion, Donald Trump was a con man, misogynist, racist, and a liar. I must admit I was excited about the possibility of a woman president. Hillary Clinton was finally going to break that glass ceiling. Unfortunately, many of my close friends in Prescott felt otherwise. I wondered if some of them were not voting for her because she was a woman. Two days before the election, the Access Hollywood tape[vi] came out. In the video, Trump described his attempt to seduce a married woman and indicated he might just start kissing a woman.

He said, "I don't even wait. And when you're a star, they let you do it. You can do anything, even grab 'em by the pussy. You can do anything."

Between that comment and the video of Trump mocking a disabled reporter, I was horrified by the possibility that this man was running for President of our United States of America. I spent that election night glued to the television. It looked good at first until the electoral votes started coming in for Trump late in the process. When he was announced as the apparent winner, my heart sank, but I reluctantly accepted the results and hoped for the best for our country!

Shortly after the inauguration, the Women's March on Washington was to be held, and I wanted to go. A woman named Teresa Shook started a Facebook page and organized this march. It was amazing how quickly it took off. I wasn't alone with my feelings. I could not find anyone that was going from my town, so I watched it on television. It was unreal! It was about the "Me Too" movement, but it also protested our new president. There were now several women with harassment claims against Trump. His misogynistic ways just added to our dissent. It ended up being the largest single-day march in US history. Half a million peaceful protestors turned out. A friend bought me a little pink knitted hat with the ears that I wore proudly around the house.

Later that year, my sister put my dad on a plane, and I picked him up at the Phoenix airport. He had been out to see me once before, but I don't think he even remembered. This time was different. My dad was not my dad anymore. He was so angry, and he took it all out on me. I tried my absolute best to make a home for him. In fact, when we bought the house, we specifically bought one with a separate casita (small home) so he would have his own bedroom and bathroom with a small refrigerator and microwave completely apart from the main house. I thought he would want some independence. We took out the carpeting so that he did not trip on it. He had his own coffee pot and dishes to make him feel at home. I put up photographs from the old days to remind him of his life. We put in safety rails and a recliner. He had a nice TV and could control his own heat and air conditioning. There was a shower and bathtub. When the time came, we were prepared to convert this to a walk-in shower. I cooked for him and brought him his food. I told him he was welcome in the house whenever he needed anything. He did enjoy watching the dogs play, and they took to him quickly, but he was so mean to me. I took this very personally. I didn't understand why he was so angry. He was not feeling well also. Since we are a mile high in Prescott, it can take some adjusting to the altitude. I brought him to the VA hospital because he was having chest pains. They said that his blood oxygen levels were slightly off, and it would take a few months for him to acclimate. He lasted ten days.

On day nine, he stood up in the living room and said sternly, " I want to go home. Get me out of here. You can't keep me here."

Ben and I both told him that he was not a prisoner. He could leave anytime he wanted. I get him not wanting to change his routine. I totally get that, but why be so angry with us? I took this hard, and it still brings tears to my eyes to think of how he treated me when I did nothing to deserve it. I would not force him to live with us. He was on a plane the next day. My sister was then in charge of him. I told her that I would go and stay with him for a couple of months here and there. We could take turns. At first, she tried to check in on him on the weekends, but then he progressed very quickly, and at one point, he started to talk about suicide. We were afraid he might jump off the balcony, and Marnie even took the sharp knives out of the butcher block. He could not live alone, so he moved in with my sister in Champagne-Urbana.

I don't know if she had the same issue with him that I had. I suspect not. He was closer with her, and at that point, he had limited mobility. He had a fall soon after moving in and was in a lot of pain, so he ended up in the hospital. She called and asked me to come out. I was shocked to see how much he had deteriorated. The doctors said he had fractured his spine, and he was in tremendous pain. His arthritis was also bad. He had been complaining for years about pains here and there, especially when he urinated. He often had to get up several times a night to relieve himself. I'm sure that he had Prostate Cancer, and who knows what else. It is said that all men will get Prostate Cancer if they live long enough. We knew that he no longer had any quality of life and that it was time, but unfortunately, it's not that easy. We had to fight with Medicare to allow hospice to come in. His heart was strong, so we had to convince them that this was inevitable. The doctors worked with us on verifying his co-morbidities. Hospice was eventually and mercifully brought into the hospital. I had been in this situation before with my aunt. It's an awful experience. Once they started him on the higher doses of morphine, it was just a matter of time before his heart would weaken. This is what he wanted from the day we took his car away. Now, almost two years later, he got his wish.

My dad had an annuity, some passbook savings, and the condo. The condo was really neglected. Everything was original. When I came in to help my sister clear out his things, I went through his paperwork, and most of it was gone. I was perplexed as he always kept it in his top drawer. My sister said she threw most of it away when he moved in with me. I thought our plan was to leave everything in case he changed his mind. What I saw made me curious about a good bit of his liquid assets. There were three of us girls, and I just assumed that things would be split three ways. I was now sure that my sister Marnie took most of her share before my dad came to live with me. It was making sense to me now. Marnie often expressed that my oldest sister should not get any part of the condo since she never visited my dad. I didn't like that. We were all his daughters, and when I think about it now, Barb probably got the worst of my mother's scorn, so maybe that's why she has been so screwed up her whole life.

I recalled my dad saying (when he was staying with me in Prescott) that Marnie had him sign something because she was afraid she would not get her share after he came to live with me. I dismissed it back then, thinking it was just a small savings account, but now that I saw the balance in his annuity and savings accounts, it all made sense. Of course, when I brought this up to my sister, she got extremely defensive. She put her husband on the phone, and they vehemently denied it. They said that he must have spent the money. I didn't believe that for a moment, but I ended up letting it go after several days of grief. That was Ben's advice to me, and he was right. I figured she took on most of the burden with him anyway since she was closer. The worst part was in the back of my mind. I wondered if she could have turned my dad against me in the months leading up to his move to Prescott. These feelings of resentment were not as easy to let go of.

The mass and funeral went smoothly. My oldest sister Barb came in, and we had not seen her in years. It was a chance to touch base with old friends and relatives. Since my dad was a WWII vet, we were offered a flag tribute at the graveside. They placed the American flag over his casket, and two young officers played Taps and then folded the flag and handed it to Barb. We decided that she should get to keep this since she was the oldest. During the playing of Taps, an unbelievable thing happened. We all saw it. A butterfly landed on the casket. Another one flew up next to it, and then they flew off together. My mom and dad were together again at last!

I decided to take over the condominium sale since I had experience in real estate. I talked my sister into rehabbing it. I can't even remember how long I stayed in Chicago. I think it was only for a month. It was the quickest rehab ever. It was a lot of fun to spend time with Marnie, and we worked well together. We painted and hired contractors to install granite and flooring. We changed fixtures and repaired windows. We cleaned and replaced appliances and staged it prior to putting it on the market. We received multiple offers after just a few days and ended up getting a lot more back than what we put into it. In another life, we would have made a great sister rehab team.

Later that year, I met up with Michelle and Tony in Colorado for a concert at the Red Rocks. I missed them a lot. The David Byrne concert was fantastic, and the venue had terrific views. It was a special night for me to be with both my kids at the same time. It does not happen that often anymore. Tony could not get away, but Michelle and I planned a trip to Europe for the following fall.

During this quick ten-day trip, we spent most of our time in Paris and Tuscany. It was excellent quality time with my daughter. We ate a lot of fabulous food and went on some awesome tours. I had a lovely time except for an issue with my bowels. I had a case of constipation after we arrived, and I am rarely constipated, so it worried me a bit. I went to a pharmacy in Paris and finally passed a stool three days into our trip. Some bright red blood accompanied it, and so I was a bit worried. I planned to call my doctor when I returned. Most of what I read online said that this can sometimes happen with a hard stool, or it could be hemorrhoids. The information also indicated it was good the blood was bright red and not black. A dark red or black can indicate that it is coming from the colon, stomach, or even further up.

After returning home from Europe, I contacted Dr. Singh. The options for good primary care in Prescott, AZ, are limited. We liked Dr. Singh; however, his office was a joke. I suppose it must reflect on him in the end. It is ridiculously hard to call the office and get a timely response back. The portal is never up to date, so that option is also difficult to use. I made an appointment and saw the new physician's assistant. This is the protocol for all appointments. Our doctor only sees us now for our yearly physicals. I would think it should be the opposite. A special sick appointment seems to me to be better handled by the physician. Anyway, the physician's assistant discussed my bleeding with me, asked me if I wanted to do a stool test, and I agreed that we should do this. She also felt that this might be hemorrhoids. The next day, I followed the directions on the test, and it said to take a sample from inside your stool, so that's what I did, even though the blood was on the outside. That did not make sense to me. Wouldn't they want the blood to be included? I took the sample as instructed, packaged it up, and sent it back in the enclosed envelope. The blood did not continue every day, and it was very slight, so I just went on with my days and waited to hear back from the test. Months went by, and then some phone tag trying to get answers, as I was supposed to get results mailed to me, but I never did. Not sure whose fault this was.

Anyway, the test was negative for Colon Cancer. I was relieved. I continued to have blood in my stool, which bothered me. So, after some time, I requested a colonoscopy. They ordered one for me from a local Gastroenterologist, Dr. Chen. This time I spoke to my doctor on the phone. It took a while to get this call scheduled, but I finally got to speak with him. He put an order in, and the GI doctor was supposed to call me to set it up. After about a week or two, I finally called the GI office directly because I never heard from them. Upon checking, they let us know, "We never received an order."

Angry, I had to call Dr. Singh's office again. After some back and forth, they finally admitted that they misplaced the order and had to put in another. After receiving the order, the GI office called me to set up the procedure. They could get me scheduled in six weeks.

"Oh my," I said, "Can't you get me in any sooner? I have bleeding and it's been months."

They said that this was the soonest they could schedule, but they would call if anything opened. No call. I waited the six weeks. Finally, the procedure was scheduled for January 27, 2019. I first spotted blood in November of 2017. I asked for a colonoscopy in October 2018. Fourteen months had passed since I first noticed the blood, and I don't know how this time got away from me. It just did!

"Not to spoil the ending for you, but everything is going to be ok."

Anonymous

Chapter 10

Shock

It was a Saturday morning in January, and it was "skins" day for us at Prescott Lakes Golf Club. A group of us put in five dollars and play a combination of a Stableford game and gross and net skins. Our foursome of ladies chatted about what was new in their lives.

One showed pictures of a new grandchild just born, another spoke of a recent vacation, and another was recovering from a recent hip replacement. I joked about my upcoming colonoscopy. It was to be my first. I had a bit of bleeding in my stools and thought it wise to finally have one. I was 59, and doctors recommended having your first at age 50 and then every five years after that. I was behind schedule. The other girls who were older than me said it was nothing and that I would be put out and not feel a thing. The bleeding was concerning, but my doctor felt as though it was most likely hemorrhoids. I was convinced of the same since I recalled my dad having them when I was a child. It might run in the family, I thought.

On the morning of my colonoscopy, Ben drove me to the new Surgical Center, and I checked in and signed off on a waiver that would allow Dr. Chen to remove a polyp or hemorrhoid if one was found. It was a rubber band that would be placed around it and eventually falls off with the lump. If any other mass was found, I approved her to take a specimen. I felt a tinge of worry when reading that part. In an operating room, I was put under, and upon waking, while still very out of it, Dr. Chen approached me with a serious and clinical look and said, "I found a concerning mass in your rectum about half an inch from the opening of your anus, and I took three small samples. It looks to be malignant."

"Wait, what?" I said groggily. "You found what?"

She said very matter of factly again that it was most likely malignant. I started to panic. I was confused and scared. The nurse could tell I was in shock, and it was obvious the doctor had no bedside manner, so she (the nurse) tried to console me. She took my hand and said that it would be all right. The doctor then told me in a very business-like manner that she would have it biopsied and get back to me with the results in a few days. Then she left the room. I was most upset that she told me all of this while I was still recovering from the anesthesia. The nurse looked at me through my tears and said that I should and would fight this. I remember her saying to attack it from every angle. I don't even remember her name, but I will never forget her empathy. Her last words were, "do both!"

The drive home for Ben and me was the quietest ever. Neither one of us could speak. We just went through the motions, in complete shock at what this all meant. I felt anger and sadness trying to enter my shocked body, but mostly I was numb. I could not believe what I had heard. Tears streamed down my face, but they were just a bodily function, like sweating when you are hot. They just came out of me.

That night was more of the same. I was like a zombie just moving the parts of my body to perform normal functions. Walking the dogs, eating, cleaning the kitchen, changing, brushing my teeth. I went to bed early, not interested in the TV that was on in the living room. My mind was spinning with crazy thoughts. I thought about my past, and I thought about my future. The panic took over my body, and sleep was impossible. Finally, I went back into the living room and asked

Ben just to hold me. We held on tight to each other, and after what seemed like hours, I finally cried myself to sleep.

The next morning, I woke up and thought for a few seconds that it was all a bad dream, but soon realized that it was not. It was real and absolutely devastating. My heart sank into my stomach. I wondered if this was how Ben felt when he was diagnosed. I began to google anything and everything I could. It appeared that when the tumor is found in the anal canal, it is called Anal Cancer. What was that? I had heard of Colorectal Cancer. Was it that? No, it was different. A lot different. The HPV virus often caused it[vii]. There was also something called Rectal Cancer. It all depends on where it is located. Wait, I had that LEEP[viii] done over 15 years ago for a pre-cancerous lesion on my cervix. I recalled now that my gynecologist in Illinois had mentioned HPV. Could this be related? It happened over 15 years ago! And why is it in my butt now? I started to read about Anal Cancer. I did not want to have that cancer. I did not want to have cancer at all, but least of all, this one. Perhaps Dr. Chen made a mistake in her diagnosis. After all, she is a small-town gastroenterologist. How much could she possibly know? Maybe the biopsy will be negative, and maybe it is just a cyst or something benign. The good news is that I never had any pain. It did not hurt at all! I got the required pap smears over the years, and they were fine. I got the Cologuard test done last year, and it was fine. I held out hope that this doctor misdiagnosed my lesion.

Dr. Chen's office called after just two days and scheduled an appointment for that afternoon. I told Ben that if it was good news, they would have told me over the phone. I knew that I needed to brace myself for the absolute worst case, but I did not know how. Ben and I met in her office later that day, and again, she was all business. She told me that the biopsy came back positive for Squamous Cell Carcinoma of the

Anal Canal, and it was moderately differentiated and P16 positive. What did all that mean? Was that the same as Anal Cancer?

She confirmed that it was. She told me that the tumor was large and about half an inch from the opening and extended back to my rectum and circled around. She measured it at 7cm. She said that it was the better of two possible cancers (Squamous Cell Carcinoma vs. Adenocarcinoma) and that treatment would likely be with chemo-radiation and not with surgery because of its size. Shit! I asked her how long I had this and was it growing fast? She said that it probably grew over the last six months, and I felt incredibly angry at that because I had asked for a colonoscopy due to the bleeding months ago and had to wait for almost two months because my primary care physician's office forgot to send in the order and then another two months to get an appointment. And why, when I went in for the bleeding over a year ago, did they not suggest a colonoscopy then? After months of bleeding, I finally had to ask for one myself.

I do remember blurting out that I should sue Dr. Singh and that Ben, at least, would have the settlement money after I am dead. She told me that I would likely live a long life because a cure was likely with this treatment. I did not believe her. I felt that I would die. It was Cancer! The Big C! No way I wanted to do chemotherapy or radiation, and she was talking about my having to do BOTH! What would that do to my body? I don't even take an aspirin when I get a headache. I eat healthy and have always looked and acted much younger than my age. I have never been truly sick in my life. I have never been hospitalized. I have never broken a bone. How could this be? I was enraged. Why me? What did I do to deserve this?

I told her I would contact the Mayo Clinic in Phoenix for a confirmation on this biopsy and a consult with their doctors, and she agreed that it was a good plan to treat at a more experienced facility than what Prescott had to offer. She tried to pat me on the shoulder on my way out in an attempt to show sympathy, but it was awkward, and Ben and I both hated her (however unfair that was)! I never wanted to see her again! She was the bearer of the worst news ever!

After just two days, Dr. Singh called me and said he was sorry about my diagnosis. I figured that the GI doctor called him as soon as I left the office since I threatened to sue him. Of course, he was just covering his ass. He said that his physician's assistant (who I saw on my last visit) asked me if I wanted her to schedule a colonoscopy when I came in for the bleeding and that I decided on the Cologuard (fecal occult) test instead (which is for Colon Cancer only and would not pick up Anal Cancer). I told him that I did not recall that conversation at all. I wondered if the PA had that in her notes or if they added it after the fact. He said we would get through this together, and I started to cry and just wanted off the phone.

The next week was like a nightmare. I crawled into a fetal position each night and cried myself to sleep. I googled more and more about Anal Cancer and the treatment of chemotherapy and radiation. I looked up the odds, which were 85%, even though I had no idea yet of my stage. I looked up the side effects of the treatment. That was the worst part for me to read about. The treatments were harsh and could be deadly, but they remained elusive to me. The side effects were easier to envision, and they were horrendous. I might lose control of my bowels and have chronic fecal incontinence for the rest of my life. Would I be in adult diapers? My vagina might close. Was my sex life over? My bladder might bleed or burst. I would experience tremendous pain when relieving myself. I would develop scar tissue, and it could cause all sorts of problems. I would have burns from the radiation which would bleed and scar over and heal to a darker skin color. I would lose all my hair down there, and it would not grow back. I could go on and on. It took me hours to fall asleep at night. Each morning I woke up, and it hit me like a sledgehammer to my chest. This was to be my new reality.

I went through my days frantically researching this cancer and all alternatives to the standard of care treatments. The standard of care treatment of radiation and chemotherapy was completely at odds with anything I believed in. I had known friends and relatives who survived and died from cancer, and I had already formed a strong opinion that I would go the natural or alternative route if it ever happened to me. I spoke with alternative care oncologists, naturopaths, and integrative physicians, both local and in Mexico. I knew that certain protocols were not allowed in the states and that some of the best alternative clinics were either overseas or in Mexico. I was prepared to travel if necessary. I investigated clinics in Europe since I have relatives in Germany. That was difficult and went nowhere because I did not speak the language anymore.

Most of the alternative doctors with any experience with my cancer said that I should take my time and not rush into any treatments.

"It took a long time for your cancer to get to this stage, and so you have time. Don't let conventional doctors scare you into quick decisions," they would advise. "Conventional treatments would potentially rid you of the tumor, but the stem cells don't usually die."

What the F?

"The treatment will decimate your immune system at a time when you need it most," they finished with the dire warning.

WTF again? I believed in all of that. I felt deep down that it was all about my immune system. The human body is designed to heal itself. Unfortunately, several factors allow your immune system to fail. I read somewhere that most people's immune systems clear the HPV from their bodies before it can turn to cancer.

Why did this not happen for me? All I knew was that I had to work on my immune system immediately. I had to kick it back into gear somehow. I was in a bit of a panic where this was concerned. I knew about some anti-cancer therapies from when I researched them for Xena and my friend Cindi. I immediately put myself on the Budwig Protocol because I knew that I needed to oxygenate my cells and absorb the much-needed Omega 3's. I took it twice a day, but I knew that I had to do more.

I googled all I could on alternative and complementary cancer treatments. Then, with a vengeance, I downloaded and read several books on anti-cancer diets and supplementation. I cleaned out all the food from my cabinets and refrigerator and went completely organic and vegan. I put myself on a near zero-carbohydrate diet, so as not to feed my cancer. I bought a centrifugal juicer online and started juicing several times a day. I was following the Gerson method.[ix] Dr. Max Gerson was a German-born American physician who claimed to have cured several cancer patients and other chronically ill patients through detox, diet, and supplementation. His work was carried on by his daughter, Charlotte. She founded an institute and authored several books. They now have clinics worldwide that practice his organic, plant-based diet, raw juices, coffee enemas, and natural supplements. I made and drank eight, eight-ounce jars of fresh juice daily from organic carrots, celery, cucumbers on occasion, ginger root, turmeric root, green apple, spinach or kale, and fresh lemon. I used those vegetables specifically for their anti-cancer properties.

I researched anti-cancer supplements and joined groups that supported my theories, such as Square One, which Chris Wark developed.[x] It is a step-by-step program that he used to treat his stage 3C Colon Cancer. He developed this program with the help of experts in various fields of research. Chris is a Colon Cancer survivor who had the initial surgery but then opted out of the mop-up chemotherapy that his oncologists strongly advised. He authored the bestselling book called 'Chris Beat Cancer,' which I read ravenously. He used nutrition and various other natural protocols to treat his cancer and then devoted his life to helping others. He juiced organic vegetables every day and followed a completely vegan diet. Chris has a huge following on Facebook, and I joined his group. I inquired what others with my type of cancer were doing. I had a challenging time finding others on this site with Anal Cancer.

I made appointments at both the Mayo Clinic in Phoenix and CTCA in Mesa to cover all my bases. These appointments consisted of meeting the whole team: a colorectal surgeon, a radiation oncologist, and a medical oncologist. I was scheduled for a consultation at Mayo for the following week, and then CTCA a few days later. The Mayo visit would be done in one day, and CTCA would be a two-day consult. They needed copies of my biopsy and colonoscopy and asked if I had an MRI yet. I said that I did not. I needed one so that they could know the extent of my cancer.

What stage was it? Had it spread to my lymph nodes or organs? I needed a doctor to order this test, but I did not have an oncologist yet. I called Dr. Chen. I had to. She was the only one that could schedule this test in my hometown by phone. I wanted to know immediately what was going on inside my body and what stage I was at. She scheduled an MRI for me at a local hospital in Prescott Valley. They called me, asked for my insurance information, and told me they could fit me into their schedule in three days. I took the appointment. They had some issues with my insurance, so I had to sign a form saying that I would pay for the eight-thousand-dollar MRI. I didn't care about money. I had insurance, so I wasn't concerned. I did not know their issue with my insurance, but I could work that out later. I just needed to know about this tumor, and the sooner, the better. I was due some good news. On the day of the MRI, I was instructed not to eat and only to drink water. An IV was placed in my arm, and a contrast solution was administered. It gave me a warm sensation throughout my body. I went through a large machine, and they took pictures of my chest, abdomen, and pelvis. It would take a few days for the results.

I spoke with a doctor from the Oasis of Hope Clinic in Mexico and another at the Euromed Foundation in Anthem. Euromed practices the methods of Dr. Josef Issels, an integrative oncologist. I asked about their experience with my type of cancer. Both places said they had some experience with it. I asked if it was curable with their protocols. They said they needed to see all my scans and blood work. I asked them their pricing. I knew that most of it would not be covered by my insurance. I made an appointment with Euromed since it was in a suburb of Phoenix.

While waiting for my appointments, I discovered the Anal Cancer Foundation.[xi] Their nonprofit was started by the family of a woman who fought and died from Anal Cancer to benefit others going through this rare cancer. Their website was a great resource for me to obtain information about this cancer and the most current treatments being offered, including the side effects from treatments. It was all about conventional treatments. Through my research, I found out that this was the cancer that Farah Fawcett had. I found the movie about her diagnosis and death on Amazon and stupidly watched it. I read that only a little over 8,000 are diagnosed with this cancer each year. It was like Cervical and Head and Neck Cancer in that they are all primarily caused by the HPV virus. How had I gotten the HPV virus in the first place? What had I done in my life to deserve this? I reached out to the Foundation for a mentor (it is a service they offer), and someone called me back. She was an intake nurse and helped people newly diagnosed with questions and then set them up with a mentor. The woman on the phone told me that it was important to find a good team of doctors and that the treatment was harsh but that I would get through it. As far as treatment protocols go for cancer patients, she called it a nine out of ten for pain, but that in time, it would heal. I was glad to know this truth going in, and I wasn't afraid of the pain if that was the route I would take. She also told me that there were a lot of survivors and that a cure is probable for most. I needed to hear that! She would be assigning me a mentor soon, and that person would be in touch within a week. I needed to find and speak to more survivors. This was crucial if I was going to keep a positive attitude.

"He who fears he will suffer already suffers from his fears."

Michel de Montaigne

Chapter 11

Fear

I kept quiet about my diagnosis for the first few days, but it was past time to tell my children. Ben's daughter already knew because Ben cannot keep anything a secret. I told myself that I would be positive and upbeat. I did not want to frighten them. I called my daughter first. I heard the pain in her voice when I told her. She had taken her grandma's death hard, and it was not that many years since she passed. I felt guilty having to put her through this possibility again. I tried my best to remain positive about the treatments and my chances for a complete cure. I told her my plans to attack this from all angles. I told her that I had found a lot of information on cures for this type of cancer. She wanted to see me right away, and I wanted that as well. I then called my son. He takes after me and is very emotional. I worried about how he would react, so again, I kept it incredibly positive, but the word cancer has a way of eliciting fear no matter how the news is delivered. I could hear the fear in his voice. When I mentioned considering alternative treatments, he said I needed to do what the doctors told me.

I thought he would be in my corner since he was such a nonconformist and always seemed distrustful of big institutions. He was, to my surprise, not at all comfortable with me going against anything that the conventional doctors recommended. I asked him what he knew about Rick Simpson Oil? He said he knew of a guy that had cured his cancer with it and would talk to him and get me some of it. I was extremely interested because from what I read, it was Skin Cancer that Rick Simpson had, and Squamous Cell was a cancer of the epithelial cells, just like Skin Cancer. My son made it clear that he wanted me to listen to my doctors and just do this in addition to conventional chemo and radiation. All I kept thinking was I needed to find something, anything, OTHER THAN chemo and radiation.

As far as friends were concerned, I canceled most of my golf plans except for my Tuesday group. I decided to confide in them, and soon after I did, I regretted it. They were mostly silent as I tried my best to be positive about my diagnosis. I expressed my need to be treated normally and not to be felt sorry for. Of course, they were sorry for me, along with shocked. They all said I was strong, could fight this thing, and to ask for anything I needed. None of this made me feel any better. I did not feel strong but rather was full of fear. I just put on an act, while inside, I wanted to cry. I also would never ask them for help. It felt odd to be talking about golf shots or trivial matters after discussing the most intimate details of my life, but this is what I asked for. I realized that I may have made a mistake coming out to others that soon. I didn't even know my stage yet, and I forgot to tell them to keep it within our group.

I thought I could handle it. I could not. Word got out immediately. I hated that. We were members of a country club, after all, and people love to talk. I felt like people were gossiping about me behind my back, feeling sorry for me, and not protecting my privacy. It was not them. It was me. I just imagined being the topic of conversations and not being there to set them straight on facts. I had Anal Cancer. Yes, that's cancer in my butt. Did they know that an STD caused it? Did I mention that? Yes, I think I had, but how had that morphed after going through the grapevine? Maybe I should not have mentioned that part.

Anal Cancer has a stigma. Who wants to think about cancer in there? Many people automatically think it is a gay man's cancer, but that's far from the truth even though it can and regrettably does affect gay men. Many others believe that you must have anal sex to get it. That is also not true. It can be contracted by simple skin to skin contact. The truth is this cancer affects twice as many women as men and it is caused by the HPV virus which is the most common sexually transmitted infection in the world. Some people would still judge me. Why should I care what those people thought? I still cared, and I just wished I had not told anyone. I wasn't ready to talk about it. I wanted and needed help, but my golf buddies did not know how to help me. Unfortunately, I did not know how to ask for help. The truth was, I would never ask. I was not that type of person. I can't tell you how many times I heard, "If there is anything I can do, please let me know." What could they do, and why would I ask them?" I needed to find people who survived this cancer. I needed to be around others who have had cancer or have faced it with close family members. Those were the people who knew the right words to say. Those were the folks who could understand what I was going through. Those were the friends who didn't ask what they could do. They just did it. They just hugged me and listened to me. Somehow, those people knew that I was most vulnerable and did not offer blind advice or compare me to someone they knew. I was lucky to have such friends because while the rest of the world was going about their routines and complaining about trivial matters, my entire world had turned upside down. Many others were reluctant to say anything for fear of saying the wrong thing. I get it. They all meant well but were simply unable to put themselves in my shoes or more likely, were afraid to.

I was not the type at all to post anything on Facebook. However, this was how my friend Carol put the word out about her cancer. I hated most aspects of Facebook. I only had an account to keep current on my kid's affairs and some of my friends who enjoyed this social medium. It was, at times, a useful and amusing way to interact with old friends, but I did not consider it a way to disclose personal information. Again,

Ben was telling more and more of his friends and relatives, so I considered it time to tell my sisters. My oldest sister Barb was a huge fan of alternative medicine and was the first to tell me about the Budwig Protocol. One of her closest friends was dying of cancer, and she found the treatment too late. It helped her friend immensely in her last days, but she could not stop the progression of her cancer. I wanted to know all I could from what she knew, and so I called her first.

Barb was also an astrologist and handwriting analyst by hobby, and I wanted to have her do a reading on me. When I told her the news, she was shocked and genuinely concerned. She said that she wished she could come out and help me. Unfortunately, she simply could not fly anymore by that point, and she was glad that I had Ben to take care of me. I discussed some alternative treatments with her and told her that I would investigate all treatments. She also did not like the fact that doctors talked about chemotherapy and radiation, as she saw first-hand what it did to her friend.

She used my birthdate and exact time of birth, along with the alignment of the planets and stars to chart my current life pattern. She often used astrology to determine when it was suitable for her to go to the casino. She felt that she could find which days or times of the year would give her more luck. She always told me that I could expect good luck on or around my birthday. She said that most people are lucky on their birthdays. As a dealer, I found that to be a true statement. Customers often won money on their birthdays. It was their good mood that made them luckier, but something was at play in the universe on that day. I had a birthday coming up. Maybe I would be lucky then, too, and this would all go away. Hah, who was I kidding? Anyway, after looking over my chart, she was hesitant to tell me much except that she could see that I was born with Cancer rising (which has nothing to do with my having cancer) and pointed out some of my personality traits that were spot on. She also looked at other times in my life that were happy or tumultuous, and she said this time right now was very problematic. She investigated my future and tried to help me with what she thought was my most pressing decision. What path would I take in my treatment? She hesitated to say which path was best for me. My future looked difficult, but she saw a path to a long and/or fulfilling life, but it was not an easy one. There would be many obstacles along my way. She asked me to sign my name and send it to her, and she would get back to me on my handwriting.

I then called Marnie. We grew apart over the years for many reasons, but after Dad's passing, we hardly talked at all anymore. I had convinced myself that she spoke negatively about me in front of my dad, and the reason I felt this was because she would talk that way to me about Barb. So, it would make sense that if she did this to Barb so easily, she would also be doing it to me in my absence. Marnie's husband has stage 4 Prostate Cancer, so I knew that she would be sympathetic, and on some level, I wanted her to know that I was suffering. Maybe I wanted her to feel guilty about bad-mouthing me. She was shocked when I told her and felt bad that I would have to go through what her husband had been through. She compared me to him. She did say I would get through it and that there would be clinical trials available if I needed them. My situation was quite different than his. I did not like being compared to him or anyone else for that matter. She expressed a desire to visit and explained that she would do so immediately if it wasn't for John. She said that if I needed her to, she would find a way. I appreciated that, and I love my sister, but I knew I would not ask her.

"Always remember you are braver than you believe, stronger than you seem, smarter than you think, and loved more than you know."

Christopher Robin

Chapter 12

Discourse

My initial consult with the doctors at Mayo was on February 15, and it was more of a meet and greet except for the surgeon. My so-called charge nurse told me that I would get an examination in his office. Ben came with me. I had asked for the most experienced physicians with my type of cancer. I met with the colorectal surgeon first. Doctor Meera had an expression like a mortician. He was profoundly serious and showed extreme concern with his facial expressions. Ben said he reminded him of the Grim Reaper. He first sat down with me and asked me how I was doing, and I said, "terrible." I cried and told him that I did not know what I did to deserve this. He told me to stop thinking that way. He expressed to me that cancer was not a punishment and that it affected both good and bad people. I wondered how many people he said that to each week. He said that I was fortunate that it was small and that he had seen much larger tumors in others who could no longer even defecate and that they required immediate APR (abdominoperineal resection) surgery.[xii] That is when they take out the anus and rectum, and you live with a colostomy bag for the rest of your life. I told him that I heard patients call it a "barbie butt." He told me to stay off the internet. He said that joining Facebook groups was a bad idea because most of the patients who do well with treatment move on with their lives. Patients with problems frequent those group discussions so that I would hear mostly bad news, and that would not be a true representation of survivors.

After feeling my lesion with a gloved finger (this is called a DRE or digital rectal exam), he performed a sigmoidoscopy on me. A flexible camera was inserted into my anal canal, and he showed me the tumor on a monitor as he moved it around. Air was blown in to expand and clear the area. Fortunately, I had a light dinner. I was comfortable with this procedure, and I knew it had to be done. It seemed like it was routine for him. A female nurse assisted him. It was important for me to see the cancer and verify that it was there because I felt physically fine. It did not look as bad as I thought it would. It was a slightly discolored bubbly area under the skin. It was no longer bleeding. I had controlled that with my healthy diet. He said that I would not be a candidate for surgery and could be cured by chemo and radiation. However, he said he would be my surgeon if I needed it down the road. I was not sure exactly what this meant, and I was afraid to ask. I liked Dr. Meera despite his facial expressions. I felt hopeful when I left his office. Later, I would realize that he was on my team if the chemo-radiation did not work, and I needed the APR surgery!

I then went to see the medical oncologist, Dr. Larkin. This was who would oversee my chemotherapy treatments. They verified my patient ID number, and I sat down in a room. Waiting was always the worst. When she came in, she had a student who she said would follow my case if I decided to have treatment at Mayo. His name was Dr. Kelson. I understood that Mayo was a teaching hospital, and this was common-place. Dr. Larkin was brief and cold. Not again! I wasn't sure I could handle another Dr. Chen. She explained that I would be on Fluorouracil and Mitomycin chemotherapeutics.

"You probably won't lose your hair," she said. As if that was my only concern.

She explained that the primary treatment would be from radiation and that the chemo was just there to enhance the effects of the radiation. I didn't like her. She talked down to me. She answered my questions with brief generalities and lacked compassion. She also seemed to be in a hurry. She explained that I would get the chemo during weeks one and five of my treatment. I would first need a PICC (peripherally inserted central catheter) line. I had no idea what that was. I didn't bother to ask her. I found out later that a PICC line is put into your arm, and it is a direct line to your main artery (like a deep IV). It is less permanent than a port. The PICC line would stay in just for the week. The Mitomycin would be given as a "push" on the first day. I didn't know what that meant either. I found out later that it is when they gradually administer it into your vein. It is also called a bolus. The Fluorouracil would be set up in a bag that I would wear as a fanny pack or carry like a purse, and it would drip or infuse into me slowly for 96 hours (about four days). It was difficult for me to concentrate on what the doctors were saying. I heard only the things that my mind thought were important at the time. I did, however, feel things more acutely than ever. She kept stressing that chemo was not the main treatment but would weaken the cells so that radiation could do the job. She seemed eager to go on to her next patient, and I was left feeling like a number.

I then met with Dr. Jordan, my radiation oncologist. His nurse confirmed my patient number as well. He was a bit more personable. He kindly asked how I was doing, and I started to cry. His nurse handed me a box of tissues. I wondered how many boxes of tissues they went through in a week. Again, Dr. Kelson was tagging along. Dr. Jordan had the results of my biopsy and explained that Mayo would do another analysis. I agreed that this was important to me. He also had the MRI from the hospital in Prescott Valley. He thought it looked cloudy and said they would be ordering another scan at Mayo, and they would do a combination PET/CT scan and compare it to this MRI. He said that the MRI looked like some involvement with one of my pelvic lymph nodes, but he would need to verify that with the new scan. I knew that this was not good and hoped that it was just a mistake on the cloudy MRI. It could not be in my lymph nodes, I thought to myself. He said that the size was too large to surgically remove it as it wrapped around at least a third of my anal circumference. Again, they were talking about the size. It didn't look that big to me, and Dr. Meera didn't think it was large either. He explained that only very small tumors could be surgically removed from this area. He had the results from Dr. Meera's sigmoidoscopy and spoke with him already. He reiterated that I was not a candidate for surgery. This made me feel like I might be at a higher stage. He explained that he would be able to stage my cancer after the PET/CT scan. I knew that I needed that scan, so I set it up for the following week. Dr. Jordan explained the protocol that would be used to treat my cancer. He discussed the type of radiation and how it would be mapped to avoid side effects to my healthy tissue as much as possible. I wondered exactly what side effects I would have, but I did not ask. I already knew some of them from my research, and I was not ready to commit to any treatments. I was not convinced that any of this was in my best interest!

The radiation would be administered Monday through Friday for six consecutive weeks with weekends off for a total of 30 treatments (fractions). He told me that if I decided to have treatment at Mayo that he would be seeing me once a week during my six weeks of radiation and then also for follow-up care.

He had dates ready to set up the radiation schedule, but I was not on board yet. At this point in our conversation, he said that he would like to do an exam. I was a bit thrown because Dr. Meera already examined me, and the charge nurse said that this would be my only exam. I undressed from the waist down, got on the table again, and was told to lie on my side. This time I was uncomfortable. Maybe because I was not prepared for it in advance, I think I sensed that this was not something he was used to doing either, at least not with women. I put one leg straight and bent the other. He asked me to keep both legs bent at my side. He put his gloved finger in and palpated the area. It felt like he only put his finger in a noticeably short way compared to Dr. Meera. The spot must be awfully close to the opening, I thought to myself. It was over very quickly, and then suddenly, Dr. Kelson puts a glove on and inserts his finger without even asking. I was angry but said nothing. It felt like a complete invasion. I wanted to cry again. At that moment, I wanted to leave and never come back. I put my clothes back on and regained my composure. Ben was in the room with me but was not conscious of my distress. The nurse was also there. Ben mostly looked away when they were probing me.

After I got dressed, Dr. Jordan asked if I had any other questions. I had written down a list of questions. I looked them over again and asked him how many other Anal Cancer patients he had treated, and his answer was quite vague. It was something like, "I have experience in this area." That did not mean he treated Anal Cancer patients. He was probably used to male patients with prostate cancer. Lots of old guys in Phoenix, I imagined. Maybe he had experience with Colorectal or even Rectal Cancer. Those were more common than Anal. I knew it was rare, so I was not particularly surprised. I did not press him on it. He seemed confident and well-read. Before I left, I asked him what would happen if I did nothing. I knew that I could not mention alternative medicine. He was a trained oncologist, and his education did not include holistic approaches. All medical doctors learn about nutrition, but it is seriously limited. His education and career were in conventional oncology and radiation treatments. He said that it would be a mistake for me to ignore this and that I needed to get treatment sooner rather than later, especially since it could be in my lymph nodes. I was holding out hope that he was wrong about this. Ben's tumor was much larger, and it was contained to his prostate. Maybe mine spread when the GI doctor cut into it three times to get the biopsy while I was asleep. I did not want to do any of this to my body. I knew that the chemo drugs would poison and kill the cancer cells, but I also knew that they would damage my good cells and wreak havoc on my immune system right when I needed it most. I knew that the radiation was going to burn my cancer, but what damage would it do to my bones, bladder, vagina, colon, and rectum? I asked if I could get secondary cancers from the treatments, and he said, "Yes, there was a chance, but not for at least five or ten years." Oh, that's a real comfort, I thought! Not! If I survive this, I will have to worry about secondary cancer down the road!

"I plan on getting a second opinion and look at some other options."

"That's your right and probably a great idea," said Dr. Jordan. "But don't wait too long."

"How long before I need to start treatment?" I asked.

"You should start within a few weeks, but remember, we have to get you on the schedule, so it could take a week or so to get you in."

"Okay," I said. "One last question. How long do you think it took for this cancer to grow?"

Dr. Jordan slid his chair my way, "Hard to tell, but maybe a year or two. The HPV, on the other hand, can be in your body for decades."

I wondered why his answer was so different from Dr. Chen's. In either case, a colonoscopy at age 50, and another at age 55, would not have caught this. I have to stop beating myself up for that. The bleeding, on the other hand, should have been addressed earlier.

Dr. Jordan was surprised that I did not immediately get on the schedule. However, he was also quite shocked when I asked him what would happen if I did nothing.

A few days later, I met with a whole new team at an entirely new facility. This time it was a two-day consult, and we were expecting a snowstorm. Unfortunately, we had an issue with one of our cars, and Ben could not come. We had friends who lived in Mesa who insisted that I stay at their house and not in a hotel. I was more than happy to be alone in a hotel, but they would not hear of it.

On my drive out, I met with a doctor at The Euromed Foundation in Anthem. They offered many conventional and complementary treatments. They work with only low-dose chemotherapy. They give you insulin first to feed the cancer. When the cancer cells open up for the insulin, that is when they infuse the chemo. This way, they can use much lower doses and achieve the same results. It is called IPT or Insulin Potentiation Therapy.[xiii] I would later understand why many patients prefer less chemo. I was told that insurance would not pay for this entire therapy but only for the chemotherapy part. That did not make sense to me at all. Why would insurance only pay for the poison? Why would they encourage you to get full chemotherapy rather than a low dose? Was it because the low dose was not as effective? Was it because they make so much money from chemotherapy drugs? I would need to do more research. I was so confused. Insulin Potentiation Therapy was the main focus at Euromed, but they also offered the following treatments:

- Homeopathic Immune Modulator
- Hyperthermia

- Laser Energetic Detox
- Ozone Steam Sauna Therapy
- Blue Scorpion Venom
- Psychosomatic Energetics Therapy
- Complementary Therapies
- Harmonic Frequency Color Therapy Hyperthermia
- German Auricular Medicine
- Electro-Lymphatic Therapy
- Bio-Well GDV Camera

I did not understand how any of these cancer treatments worked, and none of them were covered by my insurance. Only the chemo and doctor visits would be covered. I would be out of pocket for any other expenses. I did not understand why the scans were not even covered. I would have to research all of this. An hour consultation was not enough time to ask all the whirling questions in my head. I looked at their website and noticed that Anal Cancer was not on their list of cancers treated at Euromed (it was never listed anywhere). So, I asked if he had treated others, and he said he had treated a few. I asked if I could talk to any of them. He said he would ask and call me if he could find one willing to talk. I got a call the next day from a man who had Anal Cancer and was being treated at Euromed. He was stage 3, and he refused conventional treatment. Instead, he opted for treatment at Euromed. He said that the IPT therapy was working to keep his cancer at bay. It shrunk it by around 30%, and then within a few months, it grew again, and he had to go back. The cost to him was 8,000 dollars each time he went for another treatment, plus the cost of scans. He was on his third treatment. Perhaps I could take this route. Ben and I had discussed selling our rental house and using that money for my cancer treatments. It was worth about 180,000 dollars. Ben was on board for whatever decision I made. I was apprehensive about spending that much money on unproven therapies and worried that I would spend all my children's inheritance. I had to learn more. It angered me that insurance would not cover this, especially for those given "expiration dates."

I went to the first day of consultation at CTCA, Cancer Treatment Centers of America. This was a recommendation from Paul's new wife, who also has cancer. She is in remission from Breast Cancer. I first met with an intake nurse and filled out a lot of paperwork. Insurance covers everything involved in a second opinion. I was impressed with the size of the facility, although it was a bit over the top. There was rich wood paneling, fancy waiting areas, and a piano playing in the lobby (Mayo had this also). It was a little less clinical than Mayo (the chairs were covered in brocade fabric rather than leather) but equally busy.

Just like at Mayo, I met first with the surgeon. He was personable, asked me questions and showed a great deal of concern for my diagnosis. He did not do a sigmoidoscopy. He palpated the lymph nodes in my groin and performed a rectal exam so he could feel the lump with his finger. This would be finger number four! I felt a little bit like they were excited to learn about and treat this rare cancer. He asked me also to feel my own lymph nodes, and I was surprised that I had a small lump that I could feel on one side. Again, I thought to myself that if I had had this lump prior to the colonoscopy, I think I would have noticed it. I was convinced that the tumor spread when Dr. Chen cut into it. The surgeon at CTCA said the same thing as the surgeon at Mayo. I would not be a candidate for surgery, and that my cancer would be best treated with chemotherapy and radiation. The Nigro protocol would consist of 30 days of radiation and two weeks of chemotherapy during weeks one and five with the same two agents that Mayo suggested. I wondered if the two cancer centers were in cahoots.

I also met with a gastroenterologist. He was an older gentleman with years of experience. I liked him a lot. He would be there for me post-treatment for any GI-related side effects. Unfortunately, they did not have this department as part of my team at Mayo. I would later find out just how essential this was.

I then spent the night at our friend's house in Mesa. I cried myself to sleep that night, and in the morning, they offered me breakfast. They asked how I was doing and how I slept. I told them not so well and apologized for the makeup stains on their pillowcases. I tried to explain my dilemma and how it was consuming me. I told them that I was afraid to do conventional treatments. I explained that the treatments would destroy my immune system and give me so many lifelong side effects and that this cancer has a good chance of coming back. I was so afraid of going through all the harsh treatments and side effects just to have it come back. I explained my desire to go against conventional medicine and take an alternative route. This was not something that most people would even consider, but I was not most people. They just listened, and then my friend strongly suggested that her husband drive me to my appointment and pick me up. I tried to argue the point, explaining that I would continue home after my appointment. They noticed how unstable I was at the time, and they were concerned with the storm that was expected up north. I was an emotional wreck and had puffy eyes from crying all night. I accepted the ride. I had no choice in the matter. They were insistent.

On my second day of consultation with CTCA, I met with the medical oncologist. She was extremely rigid and matter of fact. She answered my questions and seemed very bright, but she would not leave an impression on me one way or the other. I mentioned to her that I was considering not doing conventional treatments. She told me in no uncertain terms that it would be a mistake.

I next met with Dr. Sheehan. She would be my radiation oncologist. I already knew that this is the doctor I would spend most of my time with, so I asked her many questions. She went to school with Dr. Jordan, and I got the impression that she thought very highly of him. Either that or she had a crush on him in school because she lit up when I mentioned him. I really liked her nurse. She was very experienced and confident. I believe they both had experience with Cervical Cancer patients and probably treated more women than Dr. Jordan. Dr. Sheehan kept me hopeful. She said I should be positive and that everyone was different, and she would treat me as an individual with a goal for a complete cure.

My last appointment was a short one, and it was with a naturopath. It seems that CTCA has a naturopath on staff. I was surprised and impressed by this. The naturopath mentioned a few therapies that they would use in conjunction with my standard protocol. One of them was hyperthermia. Hyperthermia can aid in killing the cancer cells with a penetrating heat directed at my pelvic area. He also mentioned that I should be on AHCC for my HPV. It is a mushroom complex that has been studied and has shown great promise in holding down the HPV virus and even offering a cure.

Mike picked me up that afternoon and took me back to their house. They wanted me to stay another night because the storm was starting to worsen, and Prescott was expecting a record snowfall that night. I wanted to go home, and I think they understood. However, they decided that I should not drive home alone, so Joyce drove me in her car, and Mike followed in my car. Again, I argued, but they were insistent. It usually took about 1.5 hours, but it took us over 2.5 hours. The snow started to come down heavy, and the visibility was poor, especially up through the higher elevations. They also had a home in Prescott but decided to go back home since the storm would just worsen. They even let Ben use one of their cars since ours was not a front-wheel drive. Mike and Joy went way out of their way those two days, and I will not forget their kindness.

The next morning, we woke up to two feet of snow. This is unprecedented in our area. I helped Ben to shovel. It was a welcome diversion from my worries. We were one of only a few who owned a snow blower, so we managed to clear off our driveway quickly, and we did as much of our sidewalk and our neighbor's sidewalks as we could. We laughed as our dogs ran around the backyard and made tunnels through the snow. I spent the next few days researching everything I could find to treat my cancer. As I saw it, I had three options. First, I could try the IPT treatments at Euromed in Mesa. It was a therapy that was used a lot in Europe. I had a tough time getting any statistics on this treatment as it was not used much in the U.S. Second, I could check myself into the Oasis of Hope Cancer Clinic in Tijuana, Mexico, where it would cost me 30,000 dollars for the first six weeks, and that did not include specific treatments. If I had unlimited funds, I would have gone this route. Chris Wark and many alternative physicians recommended this clinic as one of the world's premier integrative hospitals. They offered not only all the best that alternative medicine could offer, but they also had a state-of-the-art facility with all the conventional methods available, along with offering clinical trials on the most current cancer treatments available. Lastly, I could go to the Mayo Clinic in Phoenix or CTCA In Gilbert for the Nigro Protocol.

I got a call from my assigned mentor through the Anal Cancer Foundation. She was an eight-year survivor. She had been diagnosed a stage 2 and went through the Nigro Protocol. She said it was harsh but that I could do it, and it had good results for most people. She was living a decent quality of life now and was younger than me. She worked full-time and seemed quite busy, so I did not stay on the phone long with her. She gave me the phone numbers of two other women who were also survivors. I called them also. One lived in New York and was also a stage 2 survivor. She was a nurse and was two years out from standard protocol. She insisted that I ask for IMPT radiation. It was the newest type, and she got it because she was a nurse at Memorial Sloan Kettering and insisted on it. I didn't really understand what she was talking about, but I promised her I would investigate it.

Another lady I called was an athlete and mother. She used to do triathlons and iron man challenges. She was two years out and was back to working and riding her bike. She was about ten years younger than me and had teenagers at home. She told me that the only bathroom in her two-story house was upstairs and that she could no longer make it to the bathroom in time. She had to buy a portable for her first floor. She also told me that her new husband offered her little support and expected sex even though it was painful for her. I thought this was awful, but I did not comment. Other than these two issues, she told me that she had a pretty good quality of life. Her children and her biking kept her going. She told me that her dream was to enter and finish an upcoming Iron Man challenge.

I also have a friend whose sister is a nurse, and her sister had a friend who survived Anal Cancer. I called her. She was six years out from stage 2. She lived in Chicago, and after talking with her for a while, we realized that her ex-father-in-law was one of my dad's best friends. It is such a small world. She divorced her husband after her diagnosis. She said that he was the only man she had ever slept with, and you could see that she was still incredibly angry with him. She said that he was the one who gave this to her! He was a cheater, and she was done with him. She did, however, love his father Bucky. I remember Bucky well. He used to live in our apartment building, and he and my dad used to go out drinking together. I was happy that she was cancer-free, and we made plans to meet up the next time I came to Chicago. She told me this was a rough treatment but that I would get through it. I wished I could find a stage 3 survivor to talk with, but they were evidently much harder to find.

I spoke with friends from Chicago on the phone, and most of them offered their opinions. My friend in Alaska, who has two sons who are doctors, obviously felt strongly about conventional medicine. She said that I should inquire at MD Anderson. I called them, and they had a very experienced oncologist on staff that authored several papers on Anal Cancer and other HPV cancers. Her name is Dr. Eng. They had a few clinical trials there that interested me and one even included the radiation type that the one girl insisted I get (IMPT). I was informed that I would have to fly out there for an in-person consultation with Dr. Eng. I could not speak with her on the phone. I did not know if I would have time for this. I decided to send her my records but wait until after my PET/CT and staging to make the decision to meet with her.

A few of my friends spoke very strongly against my consideration to do alternative treatments in lieu of standard treatments. They were shocked that I would even consider it! I did not understand what gave them the right to weigh in so heavily on my decision when they obviously knew nothing of my cancer, the treatments, side effects, or odds. They had even less awareness of what alternative treatments were available or their effectiveness. I thought that these people just blindly listen to everything their doctors say to do without question. They don't research anything. I'm sorry, but I question everything, and I research everything! Conventional oncologists do not have such a great track record using surgery, chemotherapy, and radiation. People die from the treatments all the time.

As posted by WebMD,[xiv] five years after treatment, 47% of those who received chemo were still alive. That means that 53% are dead! The five-year survival rate was 39% among those who did nothing. This is posted by a conventional web source, including all cancers and all patients. I do not have Breast Cancer or Colorectal Cancer, for which there are millions of dollars spent each year on research, new protocols and better, less deadly chemotherapeutic agents. I have a rare cancer that uses two of the oldest and strongest chemotherapy drugs still being used. As for radiotherapy, a permanent cure is limited to only very superficial tumors. The bottom line is that radiation is strictly a locally effective treatment, often producing severe side effects. If there are circulating cancer cells anywhere else in the body, the cancer will return. The Nigro protocol is 40 years old, and they have made few, if any, advances since then. There is little to no money being spent on this cancer research. It is obvious that the industry profits enormously from cancer treatments. There is no incentive for any researchers to study any other methods. Conventional medicine for cancer treatment has an abysmal success rate, often killing the patient faster than if they had no treatment at all. According to Dr. Issels, after considering all local recurrences and secondary tumors, only about twenty out of every hundred patients can expect a cure by conventional methods. If I were to do conventional, it would be my decision, and I would do everything in my power to prepare my body in advance for the strong immune-crippling pharmaceuticals and locally destructive radiotherapies.

I decided to consult the integrative oncologist in Prescott that I took Ben to see when he was diagnosed with his Prostate Cancer. I discovered that Dr. Zander used to work at Euromed, so I was most interested in hearing his opinion on alternative/complementary versus conventional. So, I made an appointment with him for that week.

Dr. Zander did not profess to know much about Anal Cancer, but he took notes when I talked to him and said he would research things. His comments on Euromed were not negative, but they were not overwhelmingly positive either. I appreciated his honesty. He stressed the importance of getting on an anti-cancer protocol immediately. This, he said, was important for any type of cancer. I agreed. We set up a protocol with immune-boosting Vitamin C IVs, supplementation, and a myriad of other anti-cancer/anti-inflammatory herbs and tinctures. He advised me to add a mushroom complex to my protocol to fight HPV. I told him about the naturopath at CTCA and that he talked about AHCC. Dr. Zander told me that AHCC was Active Hexose Correlated Compound[xv] and was a blend of maitake and other mushrooms. Studies show that in pre-clinical trials, AHCC supplementation successfully cleared high-risk HPV in less than six months in 60% of patients. The preliminary results in a phase two study confirmed this data. He said his pharmacy used a slightly different blend. I told him that I wanted to stick with the AHCC since it had been studied and recommended to me for this cancer. He was good with that. This was exactly what my mind and body was telling me was the right thing to do. When I talked with him, everything clicked, and I felt like I could defeat this. I began the protocol immediately. I was already juicing and doing the Budwig protocol daily, and he said that was great. I already gave up meat, coffee, dairy, and sugar. In addition to the radical change in my diet, here is what I added:

Smoothie daily:

- Beyond Whey: 1 scoop
- NutriOne: 1 scoop
- Power Adapt: 2 dropper full servings to improve energy and help balance your entire hormonal system.
- Freshly ground (at home) organic flax seed:1 TBS. Put this on meals during the day also.
- Cinnamon to add flavor or stevia as needed for flavor.
- 1 cup liquid: filtered water and unsweetened coconut milk

Caps:

- Cell Guardian: 3 twice daily
- Botanical Treasures: 4 three times daily
- InflamAway: 4 three times daily
- Immucare II: 4 caps three times daily
- Vitamin DAK: one daily for now
- Zinc by Natura: one twice daily
- Tranquility: 2 caps twice daily or more often as needed. This is an herbal anti-anxiety formula that does not sedate and will help you relax and not sedate.
- Naltrexone (3mg at bedtime)
- AHCC 4 three times daily plus oral tincture for HPV infections
- IV vitamin C with Artesunate 2x weekly

I did this for two weeks, and I felt great! In fact, I never felt better in my life. I stopped bleeding. Don't get me wrong, it was a full-time job. I rarely had time to golf. I was going to shrink this tumor before my PET/CT. I was going to show them that I could do this on my own!

"Do not be dismayed about the brokenness of the world. All things break, and all things can be mended. Not with time, as they say, but with intention."

L.R. Knost

Chapter 13

Anger

I went for my PET/CT scan at Mayo. The first thing I had to do was blood tests. After that, I went downstairs to radiology and had to drink a solution. It tasted like metal, and I had no idea what I was putting into my body. I was afraid of the test. I was doing everything I could to avoid toxins. I had changed all my cleaning fluids in the house over to nontoxic. I had changed my toothpaste, soaps, and deodorant. I was now drinking who knows what, and I would shortly be injected with radioactive iodine. How bad was that?

A single CT scan is equivalent to 100-800 chest x-rays. The scans with the contrast dye containing radioactive iodine have much higher doses of radiation than regular CT scans. I was horrified by having to do this test. I cried in the waiting room, thinking about this test. I thought that this must be much easier for those who never research anything and never ask questions. They may ask their doctors if the scan is safe, and the doctor may say yes, it is, and that's that for them. How much easier would that be? Maybe I was the fool. The test itself was painless. They put you in a tunnel and insert an IV. The contrast dye is warm when it flows into your body, and you get a rush. It feels like you have peed your pants. They warn you about this feeling. You hold your breath a few times, and you go in and out of a tunnel. It's over quickly. I remember walking out of the scan room, and the door to the radiologist's office was open. There were three of them looking at what must have been MY scan images and discussing the findings. They looked at me and stopped talking. I hate when that happens. You go into a room, and people stop talking. That's a sure sign that they were talking about you, right? I was convinced that they saw the cancer and were discussing it. Perhaps they never saw a patient with Anal Cancer before. I knew that I could not ask them what they were discussing. This would be totally against protocol for them to discuss the findings with me. It would have to come from my doctor. When I told my husband about it, he said that he would have asked them.

We followed up two hours later with our radiation oncologist, Dr. Jordan. That was one of the good things about Mayo. You always got your results right away. I hear stories of so many other patients who had to wait sometimes days or even weeks for their results. How awful would that be? Those two hours were bad enough. We went to lunch and the PGA Superstore just to pass the time. At Mayo, they always verified your patient ID number. I thought that for this trip, I would write it on my wrist. Unfortunately, it was a nine-digit number, so it looked like a concentration camp tattoo. I showed this to my nurse, and she did not laugh. She instead looked at me very seriously and just rolled her eyes as if to say, "I get it, but really?" I liked her. Jackie took my blood pressure, weighed me, and asked me a few questions. It took a while for Dr. Jordan to come into the room. I also showed him my tattoo. He did not laugh either. It was a poor attempt at humor. Dr. Kelson again accompanied him. I confirmed that Dr. Kelson was indeed an oncologist, but he was fresh out of school, and as such, was known as a fellow. I didn't care. I was getting sick of him tagging along. This time I had an even longer list of questions. Dr. Jordan asked me how I was, and I said that physically, I never felt better. I told him that the bleeding had stopped and that I was now a vegetarian and juicing daily. I did not tell him about all my other the anti-cancer protocols. He pulled up the slides on the computer, and they looked like a lot of gray mishmash to me. He showed me the main tumor and then showed me how it lit up on the pet scan. I knew that was because the uptake material was glucose, and glucose (sugar) feeds cancer, so it goes right to the cancer, and the contrast helps it show up on the scan. Then he confirmed that the cancer was also in my lymph nodes.

It was in both inguinal nodes, and it was in several other pelvic nodes as well. I was so upset. Why can't I catch a break? Why does this always have to be bad news? I cried a little, and the nurse handed me a tissue. I held Ben's hand for support. Dr. Jordan wasn't done yet. He told me that it was good news that it was not in my organs. I should have been happy about that, but instead, I dwelled on the negative and asked if there could be minute amounts in my organs that the test would not pick up. He verified it was a possibility. He then said that due to the size and involvement of several pelvic lymph nodes, I would be staged at 3C, and they would have to "hit it hard!" OMG!!! How much closer can it get to stage 4?

My heart sank at this staging. I was expecting a stage 2. I knew from the other ladies that I talked with that I could survive stage 2. I did not come across any stage 3 survivors. I had to ask another question, and I will forever be sorry that I did. The friends who asked no questions and did everything their doctors told them would never have asked this. I asked what my odds were for surviving this stage. I had to ask! It was essential for me to know so that I could determine how to proceed. He told me 50/50 if I included a follow-up APR surgery and 30% without. OMG!!!!!! My heart sank again. This time, it was really bad. I think I went into shock. I sunk into my chair and curled under Ben's armpit. I could think of nothing else but dying. I needed to make out a will. I would not see my daughter get married. I would not meet my grandchildren. I would not be there to help my son or my husband. I would be deprived of at least twenty-five years of my expected lifetime. I would die a painful death simply lying in bed bald and reduced to skin and bones like you see in the movies. Everyone else would go on with their lives and forget about me. This was the worst day of my life!

I wanted to have any other disease or cancer but this one. Why could I not have a cancer that just required surgery and maybe a small amount of radiation or chemo to ensure they got it all. But, no, this one was not only rare, but it was full of nasty side effects, and they not only had to do both chemo and radiation, but they had to "hit it hard!"

I don't think the doctors knew what to do. Dr. Jordan tried to explain that the APR surgery was just in case the chemo and radiation did not work. That, for some patients, it helped them to survive. Dr. Kelson then handed me some paperwork on a clinical trial. Dr. Jordan explained that Mayo was involved in a clinical trial for a new immunotherapy drug called Opdivo.[xvi] Opdivo had shown particularly good results in a previous trial with Anal Cancer patients and would increase my odds. If I participated in this trial, I would have to agree to it before my standard treatment, and it would begin six weeks after I finished treatment. It was thought that with the Opdivo, I would possibly be able to keep the cancer from recurring.

I was extremely interested in what they were saying. I did not know what questions to ask. They explained to me that it was a double-blind trial and that there would be two groups. There would be a group that got the drug and a group that got a placebo.

I said, "What? Not all patients would get immunotherapy."

He said, "No," matter of factly. "They need to know if it will help, so it has to be done this way."

I would not know ahead of time whether I got the drug or the placebo. I asked if I could just get the Opdivo on my own.

The drug sounded familiar to me. He said that it was an approved agent for certain cancers but not for mine and that insurance would not approve it for Anal Cancer as it had not been clinically studied yet for my cancer. This trial would be a phase III trial and, when it was completed, would determine if it could be approved in the future for patients like me. I was so angry at this. If they had such a promising drug, I thought, why not offer it to everyone, especially when we have such a dire diagnosis. They told me that there were side effects but that they were well-tolerated by most patients. I said that I would need to think about it and look into it. I felt that I could pay for it on my own if it were worth it. Dr. Kelson was shocked when I did not jump at the chance to participate in this trial. He asked me why I would not do something that would increase my chances? I told him that it was my life, and I needed to research this at much greater length. It seemed to me that Dr. Kelson was benefitting somehow by my joining this trial. He really pushed it on me. Dr. Jordan then took over the conversation and said that I had time to decide and take the paperwork home and think about it. I asked him what he would advise if this was his mother, sister, or wife, and he said he would advise the Nigro protocol along with the clinical trial. He tried to explain the placebo effect, and I didn't want to hear it.

I know that the mind is enormously powerful and that patients who think they are getting a life-saving drug often do just as well as those getting it. I could not think clearly at that time, and I just wanted out of there. Dr. Jordan talked to me about the radiation schedule and that I would need to do a simulation (treatment planning) one week before treatment. After the simulation, a special radiology team headed up by Dr. Jordan would map where the beams would be directed and how much radiation would be used. It was a special type of radiation called IMRT, and the radiation curved around vital organs and was less damaging than standard radiation. It used many small beams at different intensities. I asked him about IMPT and how my friend had that done at Memorial Sloan in New York and how she told me that I should insist on it. I also knew that Mayo had it available.

Dr. Jordan was quite familiar with IMPT, and he said that he uses it often for some types of cancer like Prostate Cancer but that it was not approved for Anal Cancer, and that I would have to pay for it out of pocket. I asked how much it was, and he said that it was 160,000 dollars. OMG!!!! How was I supposed to afford that.? He said that he could make a claim to my insurance company and ask for a special request. He did let me know he had been denied in all the cases where he made a request in the past. He said that it would be a waste of time. The only time they approved this was when it was a child with a rare cancer. So, my rare cancer would be denied because I was old. I could not get this side effect sparing radiation because I was not a man with Prostate Cancer.

But what he told me next was astonishing. He said that Mayo did not charge the insurance company any more for IMPT than IMRT. It was just a matter of the insurance company approving it. What? He said the IMRT was a viable choice and that there was no proof yet that IMPT was superior. With IMPT, the radiation went into the tumor or lymph node and stopped there. It did not progress out and through to the other end; therefore, it did less damage to surrounding tissues and organs. I was angry about this. The girl I talked to from New York was adamant about my asking for this specific type of radiation, and she was a nurse at a prestigious New York hospital. I wondered how she got it, and I could not.

I said that I would investigate it and get back to him about everything. The ride home was horrible. As we drove through what is known as Bloody Basin off the I-17, I looked over at the flimsy guard rails, and told Ben that if he were not with me, I would strongly consider driving off the side of this mountain. He told me that we could do it together because he did not want to live without me!

"Nothing reduces the odds against you like ignoring them."

Robert Breault

Chapter 14

Hope

It was now February 16th, and the last three weeks had been a blur of appointments with doctors, waiting rooms, blood draws, scans, googling, reading books and medical journals, making appointments, shopping for organic produce and supplements, talking with other survivors, and crying.

I would walk the dogs at the end of my day, get to where there were no other people on the hiking trails and simply sit down on the ground and cry. Sometimes I would do it in my car. I occasionally screamed at the top of my lungs—no specific words, just a guttural scream to let out my frustrations. Then I would feel a little better and go home. I felt physically great, better than ever. I was just an emotional wreck. I had spent the last three weeks eating completely organic and vegan. I was exercising daily. I lost eight pounds. I was juicing and taking various vitamins and supplements. I had blood tests done to ensure that I was covering all the bases. For example, my vitamin D levels were low, so I took a high-quality D3 supplement daily. I knew that I was low in Omega 3's because most of the population lacks in this area. I was now getting plenty of good Omega 3 oils from my daily Budwig mix. I was on a great mushroom complex to fight the HPV virus and boost my immune system. I was hydrating properly and getting my electrolytes and minerals.

What I found interesting was how much hope I had after talking with Dr. Zander and the other alternative doctors and how absolutely defeated I felt after talking with my oncologists. I was so afraid of chemo and radiation. It shook me to my core to think about it. I went on to my portal at Mayo and looked at the results of my PET/CT. I found something remarkable. In the radiologist's report they measured the tumor as 4.5cm. Dr. Chen measured it at 7cm. I wondered if it could have shrunk this much in three weeks because of my protocols. The size difference was significant. Why hadn't Dr. Jordan or Dr. Kelson mentioned the size at my last appointment? I then recalled that the clinical trial required that my tumor be at least 5cm for qualification purposes. Could they have been downplaying this so that I could get into the trial?

I received a package from my son. It contained the RSO (Rick Simpson Oil)[xvii] that I requested from him. Before trying it, I did some more research. I found a blog from a woman named Corrie Yelland,[xviii] who cured her Anal Cancer with RSO. Of all things! I found a woman who is my age who cured her Anal Cancer without radiation or chemotherapy. She did have two surgeries to remove precancerous lesions in her anal canal, and then she was diagnosed with cancer. The doctors gave her 2-4 months to live if she did not do the recommended radiation. After reading the possible side effects, she investigated alternative options and happened upon the Rick Simpson protocol. She thought, "What the hell."

When she told her doctor what she planned, he told her it was a death sentence for her. She proceeded anyway because she was already dealing with Skin Cancer and a horrible dependence on prescription pain meds due to a misaligned sternum and Sternotomy Neuralgia Syndrome from double bypass surgery. She was desperate and did not want to add to the tremendous pain that she was already experiencing. Kudos to her. With all those other co-morbidities, she would never have survived. Well, the first thing the cannabis oil did was clear up her Skin Cancer. She rubbed it on her skin daily. Then she got off the pain meds, which was a miracle, and was down to just one Tylenol 3 per day. Then the real miracle happened. She went to see her primary, and he did a digital rectal exam and could not feel anything except scar tissue from the surgeries. She didn't want to get her hopes up, so she went to see her oncologist, and he did some testing, and sure enough, he had to do a complete 180 because her cancer was gone. Look up Corrie Yelland's Story: Beating Anal and Skin Cancer with Cannabis Oil. She even includes all her medical reports. Perhaps it's a fluke, but just maybe, it's true.

There are many such reports of people curing their cancers with RSO. Look it up. It's a lot. I immediately did the amount that my son suggested I do. After about an hour, I got super high. The THC content in that stuff is concentrated for optimal for its success. You want the Indica strains, and you want the strength to be at least in the 20-30% range. It would help if you also started small and increase the dosage. I just put a tiny amount on my tongue. If you don't like the high, you can also make suppositories with a carrier oil and use it rectally. I was afraid to do that because of the cancer there. I ended up getting so high and paranoid that I had to call Tony and ask him what he sent me. He told me to calm down and that it could not hurt me. He said just to stay home and do something "chill." It finally subsided, and I took Tony's advice to cut the amount in half. I am a lightweight. It is all about building up tolerance. The next day I did half, and it was still too much. I just did not like the high. So, this obsession faded away, and I went on to other thoughts.

Something deep down was telling me that I could not do this on my own. I was stage 3C. Could I rid this cancer from my body without conventional treatment? Maybe, but could I take that chance? I could not bear the thought of leaving my children with no mother. They were older, but they still needed me. I knew that they wanted me to listen to the conventional doctors. If for no other reason, I would do this for my children. I was leaning toward the conventional route, but I wanted to delay treatment for as long as possible. I wanted to get my body ready for the poison. It was poison. Of that, I had no doubt. They were planning to burn and poison me to kill the cancer. Dr. Jordan did not pull any punches. He said they had to HIT IT HARD! I was prepared for the pain, or so I thought.

I decided to see what Dr. Zander thought before I set up the simulation for radiation. After all, he was in the middle. He was an integrative physician. I met with Dr. Zander again, and he looked over the PET/CT and MRI. He agreed that I should take the conventional route but delay treatment for up to three months, if possible, to get my body in optimal condition. He strongly felt that we could keep the cancer from growing during this period or even shrink it.

One last step I took was to investigate clinical trials. I had asked my doctors at Mayo if there were any other trials with Immunotherapeutics like the Opdivo trial that I could enter now, instead of doing chemo and radiation. They said that they did not know of any. Of course, I did not believe them. I searched myself for hours. This was not as easy as it seemed. According to my sister Marnie, the best site is clinicaltrials.gov. Here you can find trials anywhere in the world. There are currently 363,775 trials listed on this site, located in all 50 states and 219 countries. The first thing I did was search by condition or disease. I searched by Anal Cancer. This brought up several options. Then you had to read each trial to determine eligibility requirements. This was confusing. After looking closely at some of the trials in other countries, I decided that was not worth my efforts, so I eliminated those. I searched by Opdivo and then realized that Opdivo was the brand name and not the clinical name. The clinical names were different. I should have known that. The clinical name for Opdivo is Nivolumab. I found the trial that Mayo wanted me to participate in. It looked like they were one of over 800 locations participating in this trial. It was a stage II/III trial, so that part was good. That means it has been through two other trials already and has proved its efficacy. It bothered me a great deal that it was a double-blind trial. I was plagued with bad luck and convinced I would get the placebo group. It was also clearly marked for patients with high risk (that's me, evidently) Anal Cancer, who have previously been treated with chemo and radiation. I wanted the drug, and I wanted it before I did chemotherapy and radiation. I started to search for how to buy it. I became a bit obsessed with finding it. Maybe I could afford to purchase it. I found a source for it in Mexico, and it was 30,000 dollars a vial. Oh shit! I wondered how many vials it would take and who would administer it. It was not like taking a pill. It was administered intravenously.

Then I contacted my cousin in Germany to ask her if she could find out if any clinics in Germany were using it. She could not find any information on it. So finally, I got my daughter involved, and well, those millennials know how to search the web! She found a site in Amsterdam called The Social Medwork[xix](thesocialmedwork.com). It is like the Dallas Buyers Club. The movie starred Matthew McConaughey as Ron Woodruff, a Texas Electrician who contracted AIDS in the 1980s and was given 30 days to live. He sought alternative therapies, smuggled unapproved drugs into the United States, and opened a back-door pharmacy for patients. The movie won several Academy Awards, including for Best Picture.

Anyway, the SM is a legal version of that model. It is a foundation that makes life-saving drugs available to those who cannot afford them or those who live in countries where it is not available. I am sure that they do so with the help of the manufacturers. The bottom line is that Nivolumab is available in any pharmacy in the U.S., but you must find a physician who will risk their license and order it "off label." That means that they are prescribing a drug for purposes other than those that the FDA approves. You see, Nivolumab is only currently approved for certain cancers, such as Urothelial Carcinoma, Colorectal Cancer, Head and Neck Cancer, Kidney Cancer, Liver Cancer, Lung Cancer Lymphoma, and Skin Cancer. In most cases, you must have Metastatic Cancer. That means it must be in your blood already. The bottom line, it was not approved for Anal Cancer in any way yet. That is what the trial at Mayo was all about, getting it to the final stage through that double-blind method. I wanted to help other patients with my type of cancer, but how could I do that if I did not survive.

At stage 3C, I was considered high risk. I reached out to SM through their website and found out that it would cost me 649 Euros or just under 800 dollars a vial. Now, this I could afford. However, they required a script from a physician. Uh Oh! Who could I get to stick their neck out for me? Would Dr. Singh do it? Maybe. He was the one who screwed up my order for the colonoscopy and cost me months. Perhaps Dr. Zander. He seemed the type that just might be a bit anti-establishment. I decided to ask Dr. Zander. After some consideration, he contacted me, and said that he would prescribe and administer it. I was amazed and relieved.

Before I went that route, I decided to finish my search for clinical trials. I found a few others that had different immunotherapy drugs, and they were targeting HPV cancers specifically. One of those trials was brand new. It was a Phase I/II trial that combined three different drugs or biologics as they are referred. The immunotherapy drug is known as M7824.[xx] When HPV cancers spread, they don't respond well to standard treatments and can be incurable. This trial was to see about a mix of drugs that might help.

The study only accepted people ages 18 and older with locally advanced or metastatic HPV associated cancer, such as

Cervical Cancers, P16+ Oropharyngeal Cancers, Anal Cancers, Vulvar, Vaginal, Penile, and Squamous Cell Rectal Cancers, or other locally advanced or metastatic solid tumors (e.g., lung, esophagus) that are known HPV+ cancers:

- ✓ Participants will get PDS0101 injected under the skin every four weeks for six doses. Then they will get it every three months for two doses.
- ✓ Participants will get M7824 by intravenous infusion every two weeks. For this, a needle is inserted into a vein. The drug is given over one hour.
- ✓ Participants will get NHS-IL12 injected under the skin every four weeks.
- ✓ Participants will get the study drugs for up to 1 year. They will visit the NIH every two weeks. They will repeat the screening tests during the study.
- ✓ About 28 days after treatment ends, participants will have a follow-up visit or telephone call. Then they will be contacted every three months for one year, and then every six months after that, for the rest of their life.
- ✓ Patients with Cervical Cancer with prior pelvic radiation and boost brachytherapy will be enrolled in a separate cohort to evaluate the safety and preliminary evidence of efficacy.

I was now completely confused as to what to do. This decision was vital to my life at this point, and no one could help me make it, not Ben, not even my daughter. I was the only one who had all the data, and I felt like I had to go "all in" on one of these routes. If I was going conventional, I needed to set up my simulation, like yesterday.

Dr. Eng's office called me back from MD Anderson in Texas and wanted to set up a visit for two weeks from now. I wished I could have spoken with Dr. Eng directly, but all I could do was talk to her nurse. I told her that I didn't think I had time to make this visit because it was already in my lymph nodes and that the oncologists here were encouraging me to get started with treatment as soon as possible. I regret not making this trip.

I called the Mayo Clinic and attempted to set up a simulation appointment for some time in late March. This way, I could still have time to change my mind if necessary. Dr. Jordan called me immediately and said that it was not a great idea to wait that long. Because it was already in several lymph nodes, he strongly advised me to set it up as soon as possible.

"Have you ever hoped for something: And held out for it against all odds? Until everything you did was ridiculous?"

Ali Shaw

Chapter 15

Stress

Ben and I had a vacation to Maui planned for the last week in February. We planned this last year. I had never been to Maui. It was to celebrate my 60th birthday. My birthday was not until March 23, but we wanted to go in February to see the humpback whales migrating. February was supposed to be the optimal month. We had a first-floor condominium that was right on the ocean. It was going to be just the two of us. I was hoping that we could work on our sex life, too, if Ben was willing. Obviously, I was not even excited any longer about the trip. I could take it or leave it. Most of the trip was non-refundable at this point, but none of that really mattered. I asked Dr. Jordan if I could wait until after my vacation, and he said that would be fine, so I booked the simulation for March 6. He would need at least a week to map the radiation, as there would be a team of radiologists involved. That sounded important. I asked him to make sure that the team was careful and not to over radiate my healthy tissue. I was put on the calendar for a March 18 start date.

Our trip to Maui was a snapshot of what my life was like at the time. I felt like I had a dark cloud over my head. It rained every day for the week that we were there. In fact, it snowed at the highest peaks. They said that it was most unusual for this time of year. A large sailboat blocked the road to the downtown shops and restaurants. All our tours were canceled. We planned to go out in kayaks to see the whales close up, and I was beyond excited about this tour. Unfortunately, it was not to be. We booked a big boat with a slew of other tourists. It was our only option. It rained the entire day. The visibility was poor. We saw a few whales from a distance, but overall, it was not much fun.

The trip for me was extremely stressful. Mayo was having a challenging time verifying my insurance, and so I was on the phone and the internet trying to work out why this was happening. Did I forget to pay a bill? They were telling Mayo that I was not in their system. My insurance was through Blue Cross and Blue Shield, and it was a PPO from Ben's Sheet Metal Workers Union. We had this insurance for years. Did they still have Ben's ex-wife listed as his spouse? That could not be. I know that I have been an extremely healthy person, but for sure, there had been small claims throughout the years in my name, or had there been?

My mind was racing. Not only did I have awful cancer, but now I might not have insurance to cover the expenses. Because we were in Maui, it was not easy to speak with the women in the union office to verify that our bills have been paid and that they had me down correctly as Ben's wife. While waiting for those callbacks, I worried. I could not sleep from the stress. I cried in bed every night at the hotel, and Ben just held me. I could not enjoy myself at all. The only real comfort I had was listening to the waves until even that turned into a scare. Our room was so close to the water, and the storm was growing in intensity. It sounded as if the waves were hitting our sliding glass doors at night. We expected at any time that we would have to be evacuated from the property. The weather seemed like a parody of my life right now.

I finally got a call, and it was verified that our insurance had been paid and that I was listed as his wife, but for some reason, when Blue Cross changed plans, my information never made it over to them. It was an error on their part, and they were going to take care of it. Whew... that was a big relief.

On our last day, the sun came out on our way to the airport. As we drove, we passed the area where the tour groups met for the kayak whale excursions. Well ... just to stick it to us, we saw four small boats just offshore, and a huge humpback whale was spouting in the middle of them. We pulled over to the side of the road for a bit and wondered what was going on with our lives. Nothing seemed to go right for us any longer. I mean, it was like we were being punished for something. Then we continued to the airport, and of course, there was a traffic jam on the way. Needless to say, worst vacation ever. Happy 60th Birthday, Bonnie!

After returning from vacation, I spent the days before my simulation appointment wondering what I did in my life to deserve all of this. I was sad, but I was also angry. I was in full "Why me?" mode. I was mostly angry that I had been given such dire odds of beating this. This could not be true. Everything I had read about Anal Cancer said that the odds were around 85%. I knew that I had been staged higher than most, but I was also healthy. I did not smoke. I did not drink. I was not overweight. I did not have HIV. I had no other co-morbidities. The gambler in me compared my odds to a 10-player poker game. I had to come in the top three. In poker, I often came in the top three on a tournament table of ten. I did this by playing smart. Playing smart meant being patient and waiting for my cards. It meant keeping a cool head and making the best decisions at every turn. It meant knowing when to fold and knowing when to go "all in."

Those odds kept haunting me. I couldn't shake them. I had gotten a referral from my primary care physician for an oncologist at Ironwood Cancer Center, and I did not consider this referral because of the hospital. I wanted a larger facility with state-of-the-art equipment. That is also why I was leaning toward Mayo over CTCA. But I recall that my doctor said this oncologist was the smartest man that he knew. He said that he was a close friend of his and he gave me his cell phone number. His name was Dr. Kumar. He told me that he gave him my name, and if I ever needed him, he would help me. I needed to hear what my odds were. I would tell him my staging and see what he had to say about the odds. So, I called his cell phone and left a message. An hour or so later, he phoned me back.

He confirmed that Dr. Singh was indeed his good friend. He could hear the panic and desperation in my voice. I told him about my diagnosis, and I said that I had gotten odds from my oncologists at Mayo, and I wanted to know what he thought. He asked me to send him the radiologist's report. I took a picture of it with my phone and sent it to him. He called me right back and asked me one last question. He asked if I was a smoker. I told him that I had smoked during and after high school for about five years but that I had not touched a cigarette since then. He said that was good and that my odds for a complete upfront cure would be somewhere around 65%. He felt that my odds were good. I then told him what Mayo had said to me, and I asked him how their opinions could differ so much. He said that the doctor at Mayo likely did not consider the fact that I did not smoke and that I was so healthy. He probably just gave statistics from the last set of guidelines posted by the National Comprehensive Cancer Network or NCCN. This is a place where clinicians can go to obtain detailed guidelines on treatment and statistics for all types of cancers. The stats may have been years old and may have included only a few hundred patients. The patients were not all like me, he explained. They could be overweight. They could be older. They could even have AIDs or other co-morbidities. He said that I could beat this, and I so wanted to believe him. After that day, I tried my absolute best to put that 30% number out of my head!

"Yesterday is gone. Tomorrow has not come. We have only today. Let us begin."

Mother Teresa

Chapter 16

Perspective

I continued with my anti-cancer protocol. It was important for me to take an active part in my treatment. The time I spent shopping for produce and supplements, juicing, exercising, and so on, was time that I was NOT spending feeling sorry for myself. I felt sure that I could tip the scales for myself by getting as healthy as I could. I got a referral for a naturopath who specialized in oncology. I was told that this naturopath used to be allowed inside Mayo clinic before they changed CEO's. The new CEO is not a fan of naturopathic medicine. Dr. Rubin has a practice in Scottsdale, AZ, which is close to the Mayo Clinic. He is not only a member of FABNO (Fellow of the American Board of Naturopathic Oncologists), but he is the Co-Founder. Dr. Rubin has an international presence. He is also the founding president of the Oncology Association of Naturopathic Oncology. The OncANP⸢OBJ⸣ represents a revolution for naturopathic oncology, providing for the first-time validation and standardization of naturopathic oncology. His office in Scottsdale serves the needs of people worldwide, and his focus is on children. I made an appointment to see him to ensure that I was doing everything possible to prepare for chemo-radiation.

Dr. Rubin's office was busy, and I really liked the staff. You could tell that they had been working there a long time. When I met with him, I was surprised at how young he was. He was not familiar with my type of cancer. That did not surprise me. I told him that it was a lot like Cervical Cancer and that it was caused by the HPV 16 virus. About 65% of Cervical Cancers are HPV positive, but in Anal Cancer, it is closer to

90%. I explained to him that I had a protocol put together by an integrative doctor in Prescott, and he wanted to know who it was. I figured he would not know Dr. Zander, but he did. He said that they had once attended the same conference and had a difference of opinion on a particular subject and so that's why he remembered him. He put together a protocol for me, and of course, it was quite different from the one that Dr. Zander had me on.

I decided to go with Dr. Rubin's protocol, even though my insurance would not cover any of his consultations. Most insurance policies do not cover the services of a naturopath. It cost me 360 dollars for my initial consultation. Dr. Rubin seemed noticeably confident in his abilities to limit my side effects and keep my cancer from coming back after my treatment at Mayo, so it was money well spent. He also told me to ignore their stance on withholding IV Vitamin C during treatment. Dr. Rubin was right because Dr. Jordan at Mayo did ask me to withhold antioxidants during treatment. Dr. Rubin said that there was no proof that antioxidants such as high-doses of vitamin C interfered with chemotherapy and radiation. He said that, in fact, the newest studies show that antioxidants not only do not interfere, but significantly mitigate adverse side effects. I decided to split the difference and do the IVs right before treatment and once during the halfway point. I planned to resume my high-dose protocol immediately after. I was very concerned with mitigating the myriad of side effects that were expected.

Between the consultations, IV therapy, and supplements, I spent at least 3,000 dollars in just a month. IV vitamin C alone cost me 300 dollars per bag of 50cc. It took two hours to infuse, and I was advised to get it three times a week. That did not include many other investments that I had made. I purchased a rebounder and an exercise bike. The rebounder was to help move my lymph system. It is well known that walking and exercise help lymph flow, but rebounding is by far the most effective movement therapy[xxi] for increasing lymph flow and draining toxins from the body. This was a small price to pay for a particularly useful piece of equipment. I knew that I had cancer in my lymph nodes. Perhaps I just needed to flush it out.

I joined an infrared sauna studio. I tried to go at least two to three times per week. Far Infrared heat is similar to the good heat that you get from the sun. It is healing because it can warm you deep into your bones. The studio that I joined had full spectrum infrared, including near, mid, and full-spectrum wavelengths. Each of these types of wavelengths has unique characteristics and present different healing capabilities within the body. Near-infrared penetrates the deepest and is healing at a deep cellular level. Far and mid-infrared can vasodilate blood vessels and so helps with regulating blood pressure and increasing heart rate. It is often referred to as passive aerobic exercise. Using the sauna regularly can reset the body's autonomic nervous system, such as heartbeat, blood flow, breathing, and digestion, ultimately allowing for stress reduction, improved circulation, and heart health. It is also great for detoxing. Many of the rehab centers in Prescott use it for their patients. I felt great for hours after each session.

I also purchased a Medi Crystal Far Infrared Amethyst Mat.[xxii] According to some clinical trials, far infrared heating mats have proven especially useful in treating cancer because the rays both attack the cancerous cells and reinforce the immune system. One symptom of a compromised immune system is hypothermia (low body temperature). It is caused by poor constriction of the blood vessels, and that results in poor circulation. This can often be attributed to excessive stress. Many practitioners believe that when hypothermia is present, enzymatic activity is reduced. This allows cancer cells to flourish. He explains that when the body temperature is increased by as little as one degree, immunity increases by as much as forty percent. This therapy is remarkably like what CTCA was offering, called hyperthermia. Some might call it an expensive heating pad. All I know is that this mat helped me sleep better when I really needed it, and if it could also improve my immune system, I was all in!

The most controversial, or some might say, crackpot thing I did was buy a couple of ten passes to a Photon Genie and Photon Genius therapy.[xxiii] This therapy claims: *Photon Genie is the result of decades of research and development, dramatically innovating and advancing the concepts of Tesla, Rife, Abrams, and Lakhovsky by perfecting advanced, proprietary processing of full-spectrum energy and infinite harmonics with recently developed "Skilling Advanced Electronics" to promote restoration of balance and regeneration. This life-nourishing photobiotic energy is effectively delivered by both an ionized Noble Gas energy transmission and deeply penetrating life-force energy waves.*

Those who believed in radio frequency for cancer treatment were most convincing, and I was willing to try almost anything at this time in my life, no matter the cost. I spent about eight hundred dollars on twenty of these sessions. The Photo Genie was a tabletop radio frequency device. You lay on a bed and get hooked up here and there. You hold wands in your hand, and a lighted bar is laid across your abdomen. I would do 45 minutes of this therapy and then go into the stand-up Photon Genius, which is more like a sauna with flashing-colored lights. It gets ridiculously hot in the Photon Genius, and it is a type of Infrared heat therapy plus the radio frequency. When I sweat, I imagined the toxins leaving my body. I believed that all of this, along with my other nutrition protocols, was helping my body to detox and improving my immune system to rid my body of cancer.

I thought again about turning down conventional treatment. I kept flip-flopping back and forth. I knew that Ben would support my decision, as he had already promised to support any decision that I made. I thought that I could order the Nivolumab and have Dr. Zander administer it. I worried, however, how he would know how much to give me? He would do his best to research it, but he was not an immunologist. He was an integrative physician that specialized in cancer. What if I had side effects? These immunotherapy drugs still produced plenty of side effects, and some of them were a little scary. I was fairly sure that I did not want to go strictly alternative. Could I take the chance to do this myself?

I think if I were stage one or two, I would have tried it, but I felt that I did not have the time I needed for it to work. From all that I had learned, it takes money, time and complete dedication. I looked one more time at the trial. I noticed that there was a lead investigator. His name was Dr. Julius Strauss. The trial was offered at only one location. It was a place called NIH in Bethesda, Maryland. I looked it up. NIH stood for the National Institute of Health. Oh, it was our government hospital. That's interesting. It was 20 minutes outside of Washington DC. I decided to reach out to Dr. Strauss by email. Here is what my email said:

Dear Dr. Strauss,

I have stage 3C Anal Cancer and have not undergone chemo radiation yet. I am very much interested in any other approach. I am a healthy 59-year-old female without HIV, and I do not smoke. I am HPV 16 positive. I am most interested in immunotherapy as a first line defense if possible or in conjunction with chemo only. Would you consider me for your trial? I have my simulation scheduled for this week, so time is of the essence.

Please let me know. I am desperate to not move forward with this brutal round of radiation and its myriad of lifelong side effects. My main lesion is 4-5 centimeters and close to the opening, but it has spread to several local lymph nodes.

Thank you for any consideration on your part.

Best regards,
Bonnie
Arizona

To my absolute amazement, he emailed me back that same day. This was his response:

Bonnie,

Thank you for reaching out to me. I would strongly recommend you consider the standard of care chemotherapy and radiation that is being offered to you. About two-thirds of patients who receive the standard treatment respond to treatment and are still free of cancer five years after.

Although the trial we have of M7824 is promising, only about a third of patients respond and even for patients that respond, all responses are not indefinite, and some patients do have their cancers return within 1-2 years of starting treatment. In my opinion, the best chance you have to lengthen your life and to potentially cure yourself of this cancer is by doing the standard of care chemotherapy plus radiation. If, however, you decide not to do standard treatment, you would be technically eligible for our trial, and I could consider it. But, in my opinion, it would not be in your best interest.

Unfortunately, I am not aware of any trials that offer standard of care chemotherapy and radiation with immunotherapy up front.

Please let me know If you would still like to discuss further or are still interested in doing our clinical trial despite my strong recommendations to do the standard of care treatment.

Julius

I responded again with this:

Dear Dr. Strauss,

Thank you so much for your quick response and candid opinion. I value your honesty and expertise. I am at Mayo in Scottsdale, and they are offering me a double-blind Nivolumab trial to start one month after treatment. 50/50 chance of my getting a placebo?? My luck has not been that great. I'm considering that but also trying to find a doctor that would treat me with the drug off-label, since it is not yet approved for my cancer but is approved for very similar cancers. Any ideas?

Thanks for your time. I won't send any more inquiries as I know your time is valuable.

Bonnie

He responded:

Dear Bonnie,

I am happy to answer any questions. Please feel free to call me to discuss further. It may be more helpful than emailing back and forth.

Julius

301-xxx-xxxx

This doctor amazed me again by leaving his phone number. I called him, and we had a conversation. I told him that I was afraid of going through the standard treatments and that I was afraid of it coming back. He told me that the only trial available immediately was for the M7824 alone and that he could not recommend that to me over the current standard of care. But he said that the combination trial with the three biologics would be starting very soon and that I could have some decent odds with that combo trial. I would have to turn down the conventional treatment and wait a month or two for the trial to start, though. He still strongly recommended that I do the Nigro protocol first. He said that he hoped that this would not happen but that I could call him if the cancer returned, and he would get me into the trial then. He felt that the three-drug combo offered a better chance than the M7824 alone. I thanked him for his candor.

In the end, I decided to go with the standard of care and keep it from coming back with my complimentary protocols. Just like the nurse at Dr. Chen's office had suggested after my colonoscopy, I would "do both." I planned to strengthen my immune system and shrink my tumor as much as possible before I began the six weeks of chemo-radiation treatment. My oncologists put a fear in me that my cancer would spread further if I did not start treatment immediately, so I never consulted with MD Anderson. I only got four to six weeks of alternative healing protocol, but it was amazing, and I fully admire and respect those fellow warriors who had the guts to turn down conventional treatments. Many of them died trying, but many die from conventional too. It is not fair to judge either decision!

I also decided to participate in the double-blind clinical trial for Opdivo, if for no other reason than to help others in the future with this rare cancer so that they could have access to these new, potentially life-saving biologics.

"Sometimes the only reason for us to be somewhere else is to see things from a different perspective."

Leila Summers

Chapter 17

Anxiety

The Mayo Clinic is a 90-mile drive from Prescott. Ben and I decided to drive back and forth every day for the first two weeks and rent a home near the Mayo Clinic for the last month of treatments. I was informed by other survivors that the last few weeks would be the most difficult. Ben bought a Prius to save on our fuel expenses.

Our first trip down in the little green Prius was for simulation. Michelle came with us. She flew in to meet my doctors and to help me organize my supplement schedule. I was so happy to see her, and Ben was thrilled to have someone to take the stress off him. It took us about 1.5 hours to get there. For anyone else, it would be closer to two hours, but Ben has a lead foot!

The waiting room in the radiation department was full of people. I imagined that most of the women there likely had Breast Cancer. I saw a man with his head wrapped in a bandage and wondered what type of cancer he had. I saw some young people too. When I saw a couple, I guessed which one was the patient by the looks on their faces. Some people were working on puzzles to pass the time.

When my name was called, my patient ID number was checked, I was weighed, and my blood pressure was taken. I was usually on the low side at around 100/65. Then I was brought into another smaller waiting room. Ben and Michelle were allowed to come with me. There was water and some unhealthy snacks in a corner. There were lockers and a changing room adjacent to this waiting room where I was instructed to change into a full knee-length gown that opened in the front. I noticed that many of the women had only a scrub top on and not the full gown, and the men had only the scrub bottoms on. I was the only one wearing a full gown.

When I was called in, I got quite emotional for some reason. They asked me to open my gown, and a female nurse told me that they would permanently tattoo my hips and under my belly button with tiny dots after they lined me up. They would then use these marks to line me up at future appointments. The radiation machine was huge, and it had several arms and a round chamber. I thought I would move around, but they told me that I would remain completely still and that the machine would do all the moving. I was then asked to lay on my stomach with my gown open and that I would need to lift up while they slid a tray under my hips. I found out later that most Anal Cancer patients lie on their backs for treatment. The tray contained a soft, warm material. It felt weird, like a thick slimy silicone. I imagined kids would enjoy playing in it. After it cooled, I lifted, and then after a brief time, I laid back down again on the cooled tray. They had made a mold for my pelvis to lay on.

There was a rigid plastic board under it, and they positioned more boards to the side until they were satisfied. My breasts and buttocks were often exposed to several technicians, but I no longer had feelings of bashfulness. It was what it was. I had a small pillow for my head. I laid in the positions they asked me to lay in, while technicians in a windowed booth began a CT scan and took measurements. I cried while this was being done and one of the female techs that was helping me asked if anything was wrong. I remember telling her that it was just the obvious things. I told her that I was in no physical distress except that it was hard to breathe due to my nose clogging up. I admitted that I was feeling like I might be having some anxiety over all that I was about to embark on. She told me to get off the table and sit for a while and that we could continue again when I felt ready. She sat with me and looked concerned. That was genuinely nice of her.

I wondered how many patients were as sensitive as I was. She explained that I would be in this same position at every radiation treatment and that I would need to have as full of a bladder as possible to avoid unnecessary radiation damage to unaffected areas. She repeated this several times, and so did my radiation oncologist. They also told me several times that I needed to be completely still. It was hard because it was extremely uncomfortable. They insisted that the whole procedure would only last minutes. When she told me that I could get up off the table, I asked when she would be making the tattoos, and she said that they were done. I told her that I never felt it. She showed me the tattoos, and they were ridiculously small. I said that I went 59 years without a tattoo. I asked her if she thought this qualified as a "tramp stamp!"

My next appointment was for a last visit with my doctors. The PICC line was due to be placed in my upper arm to infuse the chemo. They had to wait for the completion of my radiation mapping before they could schedule this appointment. I asked Dr. Jordan once again to please be extra careful with the mapping. He assured me that he would check and double-check all the intensities. He also mentioned that Mayo used computed tomography at each session to ensure that the beams were always perfectly aligned. It sounded like this was not available at every cancer clinic.

I spent the last week before treatment visiting with Michelle and getting my body in shape. Michelle and I worked on my supplement schedule because it had been such a huge source of stress for me. I could not track when to take certain items, how many to take, which I needed to take with food, and which needed to be taken on an empty stomach. I also knew that I needed a different protocol for before, during, and after treatment. She made me a three-ring binder to store all my important notes, phone numbers, and hospital paperwork. She also developed a spreadsheet in excel format that both of us could access from our computers and called it *Mom's Guide to Healing Cancer*. It looked like this:

During Treatment (Nigro Protocol Treatment)					
Item	Amount	Frequency	Total	Notes	DOCTOR CALLOUTS
AHCC	2 - 750 mg capsules (1500 mg)	2x	4 - 750 mg capsules (3000 mg)	Morning and Midday (night)	ck to see if the one I got at amazon is ok its pill form
Power Adapt	2ml	1x/day	2ml	Natura Brand. liquid. https://naturahealthproducts.com/power-adapt.html	
Turkey Tail (Corioilus)	4 - 550 mg pills	1x/day	2200 mg	Host Defense Brand (Current), when done switch to JHS Brand. Take between dinner and bed time.	
Diet/Lifestyle	Juicing and Vegan is great. During treatment can stick to more bland items (BRAT diet)			Exercise, sleep, hydration with electrolytes, couple vitamin c and glutamine are most important according to Dr. Rosen. Do not lose weight	
Rick Simpson	1g	1x	1g (per vince)	ROS from Vince is Co2 extracted. Mixed with organic local colorado honey. Tip of a butterknife is 1gram	Dr. Rosen is not convinced. Doesn't help cancer but helps with symptons a lot. Do not use as a suppository. be careful of using a suppository when getting radiated

Vit C Injections	15gr of ea	Fridays	1x/week	15 grams per treatment in 250ml sterile water over 75 min. Wait atleast 2 hours post radiation?	Dr. Rosen said Vitamin C injections every friday during your entire treatment and 2 more 25g right before you start.
Ozone IV Therapy		Fridays too?	1x/week		Dr. Rosen said you could do it. Depends how much you can handle. Usually dont start this til week 2 of treatment and do once weekly. Doesnt know how much it will do.
Mistletoe Injections (Viscum M)	every 2-3 days			Taking Zanders now then moving to Rosens	
Naltrexone	3mg	1x/day	3mg	At bedtime. Start now.	Dr. Rosen says to take this during treatment but if you are in pain, it may be the naltrexone - stop this before lowering your dose of radiation/chemo and see if that helps

Cod Liver Oil	3 pills	2x/day	6 pills	Cellect Brand. Cancer centers of america said that anchovie or sardine oil is better	
Immucare 2	2 pills	2x/day	4 pills	Natura Brand. https://naturahealthproducts.com/immucare-ii.html	
PLEASE DO NOT USE DURING RADIATION:	Inflamaway, Cell Guardian, Raw Zinc, Vitamin DAK, Botanical Treasures				
CBD oil	50 mg (1 dropper)	1x/day	50 mg (1 dropper)	right now using Lazarus Naturals CBD tincture (750mg), At night to help sleep.	Dr. Rosen is not convinced but if helps sleep then good
Matcha warm tea	1 tsp matcha	1x/day	1 tsp matcha		
Fasting	Fasting mimicing diet?	or 500 calories or less a day		try to fast tomorrow, first day with 2 drugs and day after. if you can keep it up, the day after that too	Fasting before/after chemo How long and what can I eat?
FULL BLADDER				Always have a full bladder during treament	
Argentyn 23 Gel		1x/day		Topically in evening. Wash off in am pre radiation	RadiaPlexRX ? might be ok to take free samples of miaderm

Sun Rescue Cream		2x/day		Never put on open wound Apply 2x daily to radiation field	Can Sun Rescue be on during radiation? NO, wash off
Pectasol-C	5g	1x/day	5g	in room temp water	
Organic Germanium Powder - GE 132	1/4 tsp	2x/day	1/2 tsp	Radiation Days Only. Dissolved in mouth (doesnt work if you swallow it). Take 2 hrs prior and 1 hr prior to radiation By Allergy Research Group - germanium sesquioxide.	
Taurox Pellets	4 pellets	2x/day	8 pellets	Start this treatement Day 7 of Radiation. Take on radiation days only. Take both doses preferably after radiation and before 6pm. Dose 1 - 2 hours post radiation, Dose 2 - 4-5 hours later	
Sea Buckthorn	1 gelcap	2x/day	2 gel caps	with food	

Glutamine powder NOW	1 tsp (5 g)	1x/day	1 tsp (5 g)	with food? Can you mix in with water?	proabably the best thing you can take during chemo/radiation
Glutamine powder RADIATION DAYS	2 tsp (10 g)	2x/day	4 tsp (20g)	with food? Can you mix in with water?	proabably the best thing you can take during chemo/radiation
Glutamine powder NON RADIATION DAYS	2 tsp (10 g)	1x/day	2 tsp (10 g)	with food? Can you mix in with water?	proabably the best thing you can take during chemo/radiation
Similase	1	3x/day	3	Use 1 with each complex meal	full spectrum digestive enzyme
Curcurmin					What did he say about this?
HPV Tincture					Never discussed my HPV tincture; should I continue it?

Immediately After Treatment					
Item	Amount	Frequency	Total	Notes	DOCTOR CALLOUTS
Mistletoe Injections				Mistletoe from X Tree. Might need to switch up the tree, as studies show some tree strains work on some people and some didnt. How do we test for this? or best to just switch every so often?	
Opdivo?	Clinical Trial?				
Long Term (Life) - After Remission					
Item	Amount	Frequency	Total	Notes	DOCTOR CALLOUTS
Strengthen bones	Vitamin D3, calcium and magnesium supplements for bone health. PRUNES. Yerba mate, and a specific diet for bones				
Physical therapy for pelvis strength					
Exercise					
Colleagues who have undergone pelvic radiation have indicated considerable relief can be had through hyperbaric therapy.					
Ask for a pat down at the airport vs. going through any machines - Less Radiation!					
Curcurmin	good to take with 5fu chemo. Dr. Goel recommends 1000-2000 milligrams of BCM-95 Curcumin and 500-1500 milligrams of BosPure Boswelia (Frankincense) daily if you have cancer. Dr Rosen: if radiation werent involved, he would say to use it. for HER iv quercetin instead. this would be afterwords				

I paid little attention to my emotional well-being during this time, and this was a huge mistake. I was full of stress and anxiety. Michelle was quite shocked to see me when I would sometimes break down and start to cry for no apparent reason. Although I had plenty of reasons, it came at odd times, and I had absolutely no control over it.

I have a friend who lives in Sedona and works at the Enchantment Village, a high-end spa that offers many different services to its clients. My friend does aura readings, performs Reiki, holds meditation classes, and gives guided vortex tours. Sedona is one of just a few spots in the world where it is said that there are swirling centers of energy that are conducive to healing, meditation, and self-exploration. My friend called me and asked how I was doing, and I told her that I was not doing well. I told her that I decided to do the conventional treatment for my cancer but could not wrap my head around it. I told her I wanted to be strong, especially with my daughter visiting, but that I often broke down in front of her. She understood completely and wanted to see me. She drove the 1.5 hours to Prescott the very next day, and we had a session in my casita. I laid on the bed, and she asked me to concentrate on a time when I was especially happy, and she taught me how to breathe.

I decided to go back to the time when I rode my new Schwinn bike that I got for my grade school graduation. I used to ride that bike down my street with my arms outstretched. While balancing on my bike, I could feel the warm summer air blowing through my long hair. I saw myself wearing a pair of blue jean cut-off pedal pushers and a yellow smiley face tee shirt. I felt free and happy. I still use this visualization when I meditate. I took long deep breaths from my abdomen like she suggested until I was completely relaxed. We then had a conversation about the things that were on my mind. I told her that I was afraid of the treatments but even more afraid of my cancer coming back afterward. Because I had done so much research, I knew that the treatment was not likely to kill my stem cells, and I also knew that if it came back, it was most likely going to do so within the first two years.

I also told her that I was afraid of having to get a permanent colostomy. If they did not get all the cancer, that would be the next step. Lastly, I told her that I thought that I had done something in my life to deserve this. I felt that I was being punished for something I had done. She was surprised at this. She asked me why I felt this way. I told her that I didn't know why exactly, but it could have something to do with my divorce. We both agreed that it was unjustified.

I tried to practice my meditation each night right before bed. My main focus during these meditations was to calm my spirit and embrace the chemo and radiation. I had to believe with all my heart that it could cure me. I would increase my odds by implementing all my alternative protocols. It was supposed to relax me. I'm not sure how much it helped. I tried, but I was pretty much a hot mess during that time.

After about a week, I got a call from Mayo, and I got scheduled for outpatient surgery (for my PICC line insertion) and a doctor's appointment on that Friday. I would then start my chemotherapy and radiation on Monday. The hospital called me on Thursday night. They said there was some problem with the surgical order. They had to cancel my Friday appointment and reschedule the PICC line insertion for Monday morning instead. My radiation treatment would stay as planned for Monday, but I could not start my chemo until Tuesday morning. My doctor's appointments would now follow chemo on Tuesday. I wondered how this mix-up happened and if it mattered that I was not starting both on the same day as originally ordered. I would also be starting all treatments before seeing my physicians. Every little thing that went wrong was amplified in my mind. I was really upset because Michelle was supposed to fly home Sunday night. I was looking forward to her meeting my doctors, and now she could not do that.

Michelle called her boss and explained the situation, and her boss told her to take as much time as she needed, so she decided to stay an extra week and go with me to all my appointments. I was thrilled to have her for as long as I could, but I did not want her to risk losing her job over it. She assured me that her boss was more than okay with it. Her boss's mother was a cancer survivor, so she knew exactly what Michelle was going through.

Now that I knew my start date for chemo, I needed to start my fasting. I discussed this with my naturopath and with my integrative physicians. They both strongly encouraged it. I did not discuss any of this with my oncologists. I did my own research and talked with other patients who fasted before their chemo treatments. There are ongoing clinical trials that assess the benefits of fasting prior to chemotherapy. It is widely accepted that short-term fasting prior to chemotherapy has shown great promise in preclinical trials. The bottom line is that fasting may help protect healthy cells, lessen the side effects from chemo and radiation, and help activate the chemotherapy's effectiveness on the diseased cells. No one yet knows which cancer patients can benefit most from this. I was told that I could fast for between 24 hours and 48 hours on my first round. I trusted Dr. Rubin as he has had many patients follow his guidance on this method. I chose just to do it for 24 hours.

Ben, Michelle, and I drove down to Mayo on Monday morning, and I went to the hospital building. There are three main buildings at the Mayo Clinic in Phoenix, and I usually went to Building 3. This time I was in Building 1 (the main hospital). I was scheduled first for a blood draw. I could have company in the waiting room, but I went to the procedure room alone. I laid in a hospital bed, and a nurse explained the procedure to me. She seemed good at what she was doing. I could tell right away that she had performed this surgery many, many times. The first thing she did was to clean my arm, the table, and her hands. She put gloves on and opened several sterile packages. It amazed me how many procedures she had to go through to prevent infection. It was a meticulous process. Then she injected a numbing solution above my elbow and below my shoulder in the soft skin underneath my arm. Then an assistant came in to help.

A big needle was inserted into my arm and into my vein. We could see all of this on an ultrasound machine that was next to us. It showed the vein on the screen. It was quite fascinating to watch. She then made a small incision in my vein and inserted a small catheter. That part was extremely painful. She kept pushing that long catheter, and I couldn't believe how long it was. It was guided through my vein until it reached my superior vena cava. Then the procedure was complete. It was wrapped and cleaned, and a plastic line with connectors was attached to the catheter and securely attached to my arm. I was told not to bathe and to cover it with Saran wrap when I showered.

Dr. Rubin instructed me to take a couple of things right before my radiation treatments and then again right after. The Germanium was to stimulate my immune system and protect my healthy cells. I didn't really understand it, but I did it. The L-Glutamine was supposed to help restore my natural balance of amino acids and prevent bone fracturing from radiation. It was also supposed to help prevent severe mucositis or mouth and throat blisters in many cancer treatment patients. I planned to take these supplements every day before and after my radiation treatments. Here are my notes for radiation days:

Daily Schedule
- ✓ Hot Tea/Breakfast/Shower
- ✓ AM Pills/Supplements/Imodium
- ✓ 3 hrs. before radiation - Drink 24 oz water
- ✓ 2 hrs. before radiation - 1/4 tsp Organic Germanium
- ✓ 1 hr. before radiation - 1/4 tsp Organic Germanium
- ✓ 1 hr. before radiation - 2 tsp Glutamine
- ✓ Radiation on Full Bladder
- ✓ Apply Aquaphor or other on Radiated Skin
- ✓ Lunch and 16 oz water plus 2 tsp Glutamine
- ✓ 2 hrs. after radiation 4 Taurox Pellets
- ✓ 4 hrs. after radiation 4 Taurox Pellets
- ✓ Dinner plus 16 oz liquid
- ✓ PM Pills and Supplements
- ✓ Bath and a generous amount of Colloidal Silver F/A Gel
- ✓ 1 Lorazepam

"If you listen to your body when it whispers, you won't have to hear it scream."

Project Warriors

Chapter 18

Trauma

When we returned to Mayo, I waited again. I drank another bottle of water while waiting in the larger waiting room and then moved to a smaller room where I changed into my patient gown. Michelle and Ben waited for me in the small waiting room. Finally, I was taken down the hall to a large room similar to the one I was in for simulation. I realized when walking how badly I needed to pee. My customized pelvic tray was on a hook in the room marked with my name, date of birth, and patient ID number. I noticed several other items marked with other patients' names, but they were quite different from mine. I thought they might have been for men with Prostate Cancer.

I opened my gown and laid on my tray, and they (two men this time) positioned the boards until I was the absolute least comfortable, and they told me to keep as still as possible. All I could think about was how much I wanted to pee. My stomach was pressed to the rigid boards making that feeling so much worse. When it was time to start, they all disappeared, and I was left alone. I started to tear up when I heard the voice of one of the men over a loudspeaker, and he asked me what kind of music I like the best, and I was quite caught off guard. Then I realized that they were going to play music for me. I told him that I liked old R and B, and he said, "excellent choice." He told me to keep still and that it would be over very quickly. The music came on, and it was "My Girl" by the Temptations.

The machine revolved around me, and lights came off and on. I faced a clock of some sort on the wall that stopped and started with different machine cycles. The beams came at me from many different angles and curved to avoid my organs and other essential areas of non-involvement. It's quite amazing. When I was done, they told me that I did an excellent job with everything, including coming in with a full bladder. They were truly kind, helped me off the table, and turned around while I wrapped my gown around me. Then, they directed me to the closest restroom and told me to treat myself to something special that evening because I deserved it.

On the way home, I was quiet. I told Ben and Michelle that it did not hurt, but it was extremely uncomfortable laying there with a full bladder. I thought to myself, one down twenty-nine more to go!

We were up early again on Tuesday morning to make the ninety-mile drive. We would be making this trip every weekday for the next two weeks, so we better get used to it. This time I checked in to the second floor of Building 3. This was the Medical Oncology floor. I had been there one time before but never first thing in the morning. The waiting room was packed. I checked in with the nurse and took a seat. I saw so many patients that were bald or wearing scarves. This made me feel uncomfortable. I don't know why. There was a counter with items that were free for patients. It looked like volunteers knitted hats and trinkets for patients and donated them. I thought that was a sweet gesture.

This was the longest I ever had to wait. I was finally called after about 60 minutes. We all got to go in. The chemo room was huge and filled with families. I never imagined it would be this large. My nurse led me to her station. It was a cubicle with a lounge chair for me and bench seating for my guests. There were cubicles everywhere with patients, guests and nurses roaming about. IV bags were hanging everywhere. Receptacles hung on the walls with boxes of neoprene gloves in all sizes, and the throw-up bags came in dispensers, like cups in a fast-food restaurant. There were tables full of snacks and a vending area with coffee and cold beverages. Some stations were bigger than others, and some were private rooms with beds. My nurse checked my ID number and asked for my name and birthdate. I imagined that in a place this large, there actually could be someone with the same name and birthdate. They also checked my wristband, which was given to me at check-in. They ordered the drugs, and we waited again. After about 45 minutes, they put heparin in my PICC line to make sure I would have no clotting.

The nurse then gave me some information on the first chemotherapeutic agent, 5-Fluorouracil or Five-FU, for short. I had since learned that patients jokingly referred to this drug as "five feet under" because it is so toxic. It is a pyrimidine analogue classified as an antimetabolite. It is used for various cancers, including breast, colon, rectal, pancreatic, and stomach. Five-FU incorporates into RNA and can result in major effects on both RNA processing and functions. I would find out later just how toxic this drug can be. The nurse put on a gown and gloved up before handling it. First, she injected pre-medications into my line. She explained that these were anti-nausea medications. Next, she told me that I would be seeing Dr. Kelson before I left the chemo area as he would be bringing me a script for additional anti-nausea meds that I could fill on my way home.

I would need to take those before the ones that she was giving me wore off. I felt a little funny after the meds were given to me. She then hooked up a bag and attached it to my PICC line. There was long tubing that was attached to the bag. The chemo would go into me by slow drip for a 96-hour cycle. She instructed me on how to care for myself while wearing the bag. I was not to bathe, only shower. I could not unhook it for any reason. If it came loose or undone, the unit would sound an alarm, and I would immediately need to go to the ER. If the alarm went off and it was just a kink in the line, it would stop when I unkinked it. I was warned to flush twice after I urinated because of the toxicity. *Really*? The machine made a little noise when it pumped into me and then stopped when it was done. It had a timer on it that showed how many hours and minutes were left. A black faux leather case held the bag, and I had a choice to wear it as a fanny pack or a shoulder bag. I chose the shoulder bag. No way I was going to look like an old lady with a fanny pack! Then Dr. Kelson showed up and asked how things were going. I said fine but commented on how long everything took. He asked if I had any questions, and I did not. He then gave me the scripts for the anti-nausea meds and left.

The nurse came in again, and now she was putting on another fresh gown and gloves to give me my push of Mitomycin. It was a huge vial of purple liquid. I thought of windshield washer solvent when I saw it. By hand, she slowly pushed the liquid into my vein. It must have taken 20 minutes. I couldn't believe that there was no better way to do this! I was terrified, thinking about all this poison being put into my body and what it might do to me.

We left with all our instructions. My next visit was with Dr. Jordan. He asked me how my first radiation treatment was, and I told him it went well and that I liked the techs. He agreed that they were the best of the best. He told me that I would see him weekly from now until the end of treatment. I would see him every Friday afternoon at one pm. He explained how they would be radiating all my pelvic lymph nodes, with the main tumor site receiving the highest dose. The total amount of radiation would be 54Gy or gray. This is the absorbed dose of ionizing radiation. My radiation appointments would be at 11 am every day. This way, I would not have to deal with traffic coming from or going back to Prescott. I appreciated that the schedule would allow for this and told him that soon I would be moving to Cave Creek to make the commute easier as side effects became tougher. He agreed that this would be a good idea as the radiation treatments took time to start working, and in the later weeks, I could expect more discomfort in terms of redness and pain, especially when urinating or defecating. I would also potentially get urgent diarrhea. Some patients did, and others did not, but that I should be prepared for it. His nurse gave me a whole bag of Aquaphor samples. She told me to put this on immediately after radiation to help with the burning and dryness. She also gave me a blow-up pad to sit on when it got too uncomfortable. She said it would be a good idea for me to bring this with me wherever I went. I left the office thinking, *Oh my, what did I get myself into?*

We stopped for a bite to eat, and by the time we got home, it was already dark, and I was exhausted. I laid down to rest and accidentally fell asleep. Ben went to the pharmacy and got my prescriptions filled. He didn't want to wake me. In the middle of the night, I woke up feeling extremely nauseous. I found the pills that Ben had gotten for me, and I took them immediately. I laid back down, but the nausea just got worse and worse. I became increasingly ill and threw up. I felt a little better for a few minutes and then got sick again. I could not stop throwing up. By then, the whole house was up. Ben and Michelle did not know what to do for me, and I could not keep anything down. I tried to drink water to stay hydrated, but I would just throw it up. Hours went by, and I tried to take another pill. That would not stay down either. How was I going to take my pill or drink water if I could not keep anything down? I had never been this sick to my stomach in my entire life. It was worse than food poisoning. I had food poisoning once and stomach flu a few times, but nothing like this. Finally, Ben called the number they gave us for Mayo. It was an after-hours number, and so we got the physician on call. He said to go to the ER if I did not stop throwing up and get something by

IV. I tried to sleep and just kept dry heaving. Finally, we decided that I needed to go to the ER. At the ER, we waited for about an hour, and then I got some IV anti-nausea meds that seemed to help a little. They also gave me IV hydration. I was still extremely ill, and it was already the next morning. I wondered how we would ever make it to our radiation appointment, so we called Dr. Jordan, expecting to cancel.

He said that I needed to go. He said that if we could not go by car, he would arrange for an ambulance to take me from the hospital in Prescott to the Mayo Clinic in Phoenix. We thought, OMG, they really are serious about not missing a radiation treatment. Well, we packed up our belongings and stopped home to freshen up, and off we were again to my radiation session. We made it in time for my session, and, with all the commotion, my bladder was not full. They brought me another bottle of water and told me to drink it and took other patients ahead of me. I just wanted to get it over with, but I had a tough time drinking the water. It made me sick.

I hated that bag of poison that kept going into me. The machine beeped every time I fell asleep on the line, and I had to unkink it. I hated everything about it. Finally, they took me in and said that I was okay to get the radiation treatment, and I thought to myself that my bladder was not full enough. They said it was okay to do it a couple of times when my bladder was not full but not to make a habit of it. I did not like it, but everyone was waiting for me, so I went ahead with the radiation even though my bladder was not full. They could see by the computed tomography (CT) that it was about 60 percent of where they like it to be. Yesterday I was at 100%!

I had the same two techs and learned that their names were John and Eric. John was a shorter man who walked with a little limp. I wanted to ask him why he limped, but I did not. Eric was taller and had dark hair. Both were probably in their thirties. They knew that I had come straight from the ER and that I was not feeling well. They told me that if I needed to throw up, just to let them know, and they could stop the process at any time. I was grateful for that because I felt like shit. We got through it, and I promised myself that I would never let this happen again where my bladder was not full for radiation. I also knew that I could not chance taking my anti-nausea pills late.

That night I took a Lorazepam to help me sleep. It was one of the other drugs that Dr. Kelson gave me a prescription for. He also gave me Hydrocodone which I planned to stay away from. I knew all about that drug, and I wanted no part of it. The next day, I still felt sick. Not as bad as the first, but still really sick. I threw up again. I tried my best to keep drinking water. I ate a couple of crackers too. I also tried to keep on my anti-nausea medications. Unfortunately, they were not working very well. Why was I having such an issue with these chemo drugs? Chemo hated me, and I hated it! I went to Mayo again, and the ride there was awful. I just reclined my seat and tried not to feel the bumps and turns. The Prius was not like our Lexus. I was glad we were saving money, but right then, I wished I was in the comfort of our Lexus and not in this bumpy green hornet.

This time my bladder was at 80% when they took me in. They said it was fine. They just did not want it to ever be below 60%. I thought to myself that 100% would be better. *Why could I not achieve this?* I was disappointed in myself. I was also quite disappointed that I could not take any of my supplements or do my juicing. It caused me a great deal of anxiety. Michelle was leaving that night, and so we took her to the airport after my radiation treatment. It was sad to see her leave. She said that she would come back during my second to last week and stay with me in Cave Creek so that Ben could have a break and golf with his friends on their yearly trip. I was looking forward to that.

That night I started to feel extremely sick again. I was itchy too. Again, I could not keep down my pills or any liquids, so off we went to the ER again. This time, we went earlier than the last time because we knew that Mayo would still want me to go to radiation the next morning. We waited for over two hours this time. While I was waiting, I threw up a couple of times. I was always amazed at the other people in the waiting room. Some came in with obvious heart problems, and they were taken in immediately. Some looked like they were looking for pain meds, and some had obvious burns or broken bones. Still, others had breathing problems and came in with their oxygen tanks. When I finally got a bed, they hooked me up to IV hydration again, and since my rash was getting much worse, they gave me IV Phenergan. I knew the nurse this time. It was a small town, and I had played Bunco with her a few times in the past. The staff was kind at Yavapai Hospital.

Phenergan was not helping. I think it did help, however, to get the hydration. I got two bags this time. I also got more of the IV anti-nausea drugs. We called Dr. Kelson from the hospital. He seemed surprised that I was there again. I told him that I could not keep fluids down and that I was developing this itchy rash and even had swelling in my hands. He did not like that they gave me IV Phenergan at the hospital and felt that I might have reacted to that. He wanted me on Benadryl. I told him that the rash started before that, and that's why they gave it to me. This made absolutely no sense to me. I also wanted to know why the anti-nausea meds were not working for me. Lastly, I asked him if he could schedule hydration for me at Mayo during the four days that I was on the Five FU so that I did not end up in the Emergency Room every night.

I wanted to talk to Dr. Larkin (the medical oncologist that was supposed to be on my "team,") but Dr. Kelson said she was out of town. He explained that he would call her and ask her opinion on all of it. I wondered how long that would take. Why was I saddled with this inexperienced oncologist for something this vital? I needed some answers, and I needed them now. We came home late that night and got a few hours of sleep before driving to Phoenix again. I did not hear back from Dr. Kelson. He said that he would order the hydration for me, but I had no idea when. I watched the timer on my bag, and I could not wait to have this thing off me. I can't tell you how many times I just wanted to rip the bag off. The skin on my neck was so thick from the hives, and I had no answers on what to do about it. Today was Friday, so I was due to meet with Dr. Jordan. I hoped he would have an answer for me because Benadryl wasn't doing a thing. I was beyond miserable.

John and Eric were there again for my treatment, and they said that my bladder was at 70 percent. Again, I did my best to drink as much water as I could. I was stressed again, thinking that my bladder was not as full as it should be, but I did not want to go back to the waiting room, and I had other appointments that I needed to get to today. John told me not to worry. He said that starting Monday, I would be off the chemo bag, and I could make up for it. He reiterated that it only needed to be above 60%.

I then went to the Oncology floor for my hydration and to have my Five FU bag and PICC line removed. There were still two hours left on the chemo bag, so they said that I had to return after my appointment with Dr. Jordan, and there was no order put in for hydration. I was so disappointed.

At my appointment with Dr. Jordan, I told him how unhappy I was with the Medical Oncology Dept. He looked at

Jackie and then said that this was not the first time he had heard this. I told him that I had been to the ER twice for dehydration and the rash and that I could not stop throwing up. When I needed answers about chemotherapy's side effects, I told him that I should not have to wait for Dr. Kelson to phone Dr. Larkin. I showed him the rash and told him what Kelson had said to me. He saw how bad it was and noted the circular welts and prescribed a course of steroids for me. He said that it was from the chemo. That's what I thought! He agreed that it was a good idea for me to get daily hydration during my chemotherapy weeks and that he would make sure it got ordered for the next round. He was unsure why the anti-nausea meds were not working but assured me that it would be better once I was off the bag. He looked at my pelvic area. It was just slightly red. He prepared me for what would come with the next few weeks of treatment. He said that I would need to start applying the Aquaphor ointment right after my treatments from now on. He said that I would lose all my hair down there and that it would burn and peel like a bad sunburn, especially in the soft area at my inguinal canal (groin).

I checked in again, and it took me over an hour to get called. Finally, they unhooked my bag. Thank God that awful poison was finished. Unfortunately, it was now somewhere in my body wreaking havoc. I had no idea how I would do this again in week five. The mere thought of it made me sick to my stomach.

My rash started to improve almost immediately upon starting the steroids. I left a long message to Dr. Kelson on his portal. This way, there would be a record of it. Here is what I said:

Dear Dr. Kelson,

I had several concerns when we spoke last Thursday. Do you recall that conversation? You were going to call me right back. It is now Wednesday. We also discussed my getting hydration therapy and dissolvable or IV anti-nausea drugs during my next chemo round. I got a call this Monday after my radiation treatment from a scheduler that said you ordered hydration for me that day. I don't understand. I told her that must be a mistake?? I was done with chemo already.

As you probably know, I am not happy with Mayo's decision to have me consult with a seasoned medical oncologist and then have me actually treated by a fellow/resident and never see that oncologist again. Her name is on my portal, as though I have the ability to consult with her, yet I do not. She is supposed to be on my "team," and my team is supposed to discuss my case weekly. I have several issues with my treatment so far and am discussing them with Mayo's Patient Experience Department. I am also consulting with outside medical oncology care.

I am not angry. I am just advocating for myself. I don't have the energy to be angry, nor will it serve me well at this time when I am fighting for my life.

Regards,
Bonnie L

I am sure that Dr. Kelson was not happy after reading this message, but I felt desperate for answers to my concerns. I know he is an oncologist, but he has zero practical experience. So, I had to consult with Dr. Kumar in person after my first chemo round. He is an oncologist that is good friends with Dr. Singh. He told me the rash was definitely caused by the 5FU, not the Phenergan, and agreed with Dr. Jordan that I should be treated with Medrol. He also told me that when his patients do not tolerate or cannot be helped with the standard anti-nausea drugs of Compazine and Zofran, he gives them an IV cocktail of Aloxi and Amend. He said that I should ask for these in my next round and call him anytime I needed. It was a comfort to have him in my back pocket, but it was frustrating that Mayo did not have a competent medical oncologist on my so-called "team!"

The next week, I developed chest pain. I did not know what this was. I called Dr. Kelson because I felt it was related to the chemo. He said he would call me back. It took him another day. For chest pain, it took him a day! It got a bit better, so I just let it go, but I was pissed. He finally called me back and put me on Zantac for heartburn. He said that it would take time for the Zantac to start working. He also gave me a prescription for Lorazepam which helped more than the Zantac because it made me sleepy, and with sleep, I was not in pain. The rash subsided with the steroid pack from Dr. Jordan. I then developed some mild mouth sores, for which I was prescribed a Lidocaine rinse.

My radiation treatments started to produce diarrhea, so I was put on Lomotil for that. I was starting to have a challenging time eating. Nothing tasted right, and I had no appetite. I was warned of this. Ben cooked oatmeal or scrambled eggs for breakfast and usually some soup and crackers for lunch. I often fell asleep before dinner and woke up several times during the night. I could tell that I was losing weight, but I was not concerned about it. I remember someone telling me to be careful not to lose too much weight, but I never imagined needing to be concerned about my weight. I always had a good appetite and had plenty of extra meat on my bones.

This was the last week that we would have to make the long drive to Phoenix. This was also my Birthday week. Woo-hoo!!!!! I was turning sixty. I remember a friend of mine turned sixty, and her significant other gave her a big surprise party at the club. It was a great celebration. I would celebrate my 60th birthday with a radiation treatment and a Lorazepam. I would dream of happier days when I was a fearless young girl, riding my bike on a warm summer day without a care in the world.

On Sunday, we left for the Cave Creek casita, where we would spend the next month. Many of our friends stopped by to say goodbye and offered to help with the dogs. However, we had already decided to bring them with us. My friends and family called and texted me during my treatment. One girl I played golf with occasionally took note of my start date and sent me a daily text with an inspirational quote and a joke. I was wondering to myself when she would tire of this, but she sent one every day. Here is an example:

> *Inspirational: To be honest with you, I don't have the words to make you feel better, but I do have the arms to give you a hug, ears to listen to whatever you want to talk about, and I have a heart; a heart that's aching to see you smile again.*

> *Joke: A hacker spends a day at a plush country club, playing golf and enjoying the luxury of a complimentary caddy. Being a hacker, he, of course, plays poorly all day. Round about the 18th hole, he spots a lake off the left of the fairway. He looks at the caddy and says, "I've played so lousy all day, I think I'm going to go drown myself in that lake." The caddy looks back at him and says, "I don't think you could keep your head down that long."*

I really looked forward to reading her texts, and I will never forget this special gift from an incredibly special friend.

The Cave Creek casita was a perfect location. The owner lived on the property with his wife and two teenaged daughters. He was a contractor, and his wife was a nurse. They knew that I was going to the Mayo Clinic every day for radiation, and they were very accommodating to all our needs.

We were in a separate building just behind the main house. It was very private and completely remodeled. It had a full kitchen/living room area with a big-screen TV and pull-out sofa. The bedroom had an amazingly comfortable queen-sized bed and a small private bath. The only thing I worried about was that there was no bathtub. I also wished that there was a television in the bedroom. I like to watch TV in bed. Ben went out that same day and bought one, and he and the owner hooked it up. It was so thoughtful.

The dogs took some time to get used to the place. They were a bit of a pain because they wanted to go out all the time. At home, they were in and out constantly, but here we could not let them out into the yard. It was fenced, but the owners had a small dog, and our dogs are not that friendly! We had to walk them twice a day, and it was ridiculously hot outside. I didn't mind that much. I was always cold since my treatment started. The dogs would occasionally get cactus needles stuck in their paws on the walks, so we had to pull them out with tweezers. After a time, we wished we had gotten a sitter and left them home.

Week three of treatment was my easiest week in some ways. I did start to experience more fatigue and more mouth sores. I continued to have a tough time eating. Ben did his best to cook for me, but his skills were limited. We were looking forward to Michelle's visit the next week, and Tony was coming a few days later, so it would be extra special to have them both with me. They are both excellent cooks. Ben planned to go back to Prescott that week, and he would take the dogs with him.

Toward the end of week three, I started to lose my hair. I was surprised because that was the one thing that Dr. Larkin had said would not happen. At first, I would find extra hair in my brush. Then after I shampooed my hair, it would come out in clumps in my hands. I wasn't prepared for the emotional toll it took on me. It was so depressing to have this happen. I would wake up in the morning and find hair all over my pillow. I was afraid to brush my hair for fear that it would all come off.

We picked up Michelle at the airport on a Saturday. It was great to have her there. She slept on the hideaway, and Ben stayed one more night with me. Then, he left for Prescott on Sunday with the dogs.

On Monday of week four, Michelle went with me to my radiation treatment. After treatment, we went up to the Oncology floor, where there was a salon with wigs, scarves, and hats. I decided to have my head shaved. I couldn't stand it any longer! I hated having it fall out. The girl who would cut my hair asked me how long I wanted it, and I told her to get rid of it all. She asked me if I was sure, and I said that I was. Michelle watched as I had my entire scalp buzzed. It was a melancholy feeling. Now I was truly 'the girl with cancer.' My head wasn't as bumpy as I thought it would be, but I immediately purchased a pretty scarf and tried on a few wigs. My head was cold! When we left, she told us about another salon down the road that was much larger, so we went there straight away. There was no charge for the buzz cut. I tried to leave a tip, but she would not take it.

At the Wig Shop, I tried on several wigs. It was kind of fun. I tried on a long curly pink wig and several blonde wigs of all different lengths and styles. We took pictures and sent them to some friends. I tried on some that were even connected to hats or scarves. I liked several. I found out that my insurance covered 500 dollars, so I spent every bit of that amount on two wigs. I wore my wigs to treatment every day that week and my doctor's appointment on Friday also.

By the middle of week four, I was starting to feel the effects of the radiation. My hair fell out from my pubic area, and the delicate skin in all my private areas began to feel like a bad sunburn. I thought, wow, my first full Brazilian! It hurt to sit, and it hurt to relieve myself. I was uncomfortable in my regular clothes, so I started to wear more skirts and loose-fitting shorts. At the same time, the fatigue from chemo hit me. This was one thing that Dr. Kelson got right. He told me that in week four, my white blood cell count would drop considerably, and I would experience extreme fatigue. I would be getting a full set of labs soon to ensure that they did not drop too low. When that happens, it is called Neutropenia. If I got a bad case of that, they would have to withhold my second chemo regime, and I would be susceptible to any infection.

My son was due to come in, and I was too tired to go to the airport to meet him. Michelle picked him up. We had a nice visit that night, and they cooked dinner for me. I ate what I could, but nothing tasted right anymore, and my appetite was dwindling. Mostly I laid in bed. I noticed that night that I now had hips like a boy. I always had a full figure, especially in my hips. I couldn't believe I had lost weight from this area of my body. My stomach was also completely flat. I can't remember the last time I had a flat stomach. I figured I would gain it back after treatment ended. I wondered how I looked to my kids. It must have frightened them to see me so weak, thin, and bald. Ben came back the day that Michelle was due to leave. I hated to see her go, but I also did not want her there for my last two weeks. I knew that chemo did not like me, and I also knew from speaking to other survivors, that the burns would get much worse.

On Friday of week four, I had my radiation treatment, and for the first time, I did not have John and Eric. I was in another room with two women. I asked them where my boys were, and they said they would take good care of me. They were also genuinely nice to me. We worked hard to keep my bladder over 60%. After my treatment, one of the female techs asked me if I had seen the People magazine in the waiting room, and I said that I had not. She told me that there was a feature story about Marcia Cross. Marcia Cross is the redhead from Desperate Housewives.

"She was diagnosed with Anal Cancer over a year ago and is coming out now to share her story."

"Really?" I asked her. "I will have to read about it. Thanks."

After getting dressed, I found the magazine and sat down with it. First Farah Fawcett and now Marcia Cross. The article said that she went through chemo-radiation last year and now wants to bring awareness to this rare cancer and fight some of its stigma. I teared up reading the article. She called the treatments "gnarly" and said that she wants the shame surrounding Anal Cancer to stop! There were pictures of her bald, but of course, she looked great. I was glad she survived and glad she came out about it.

I was more than half done with my Nigro protocol, and Dr. Rubin thought this would be a suitable time for me to do a vitamin C IV. I did not get approval from Dr. Jordan or Dr. Kelson for this. In fact, they instructed me not to do any antioxidants during Chemo. Well, this was not during chemo. This was as far away from chemo as I could get.

My appointment with Dr. Rubin was on Friday afternoon after radiation and before my appointment with Dr. Jordan. I was hungry after radiation, and so was Ben. He wanted Portillo's, so we stopped there. I decided to have their pasta with marinara sauce. How bad could that be? I ate about half of it. Ben dropped me off at Dr. Rubin's office, where I was hooked up to my IV. I sat there with two other patients. He always had a full schedule. We talked about our cancers. We discussed books and supplements. The woman next to me was fighting stage 4 Cervical Cancer. It was a cancer that is remarkably similar to mine. We had an immediate connection. She was very thin, like me, but had so much more energy. She was "all in" on her naturopathic protocol. She was through with conventional cancer treatments but did not pass judgment on me. She had "been there" and "done that." She simply had no use for them any longer. She struck me as very feisty and had an air of confidence. She asked a lot of questions from the staff, and they all knew her well. I took it that she was a "regular." She asked me a lot of questions too. Her goal seemed to be to find out what was working for me and what she could learn from it.

On the other hand, she was also empathetic toward my situation but optimistic toward my recovery. She did not feel sorry for me. My new IV friend had what some would describe as the "will to live," and she somehow projected this "will" onto me. We were both getting high-dose vitamin C, so we talked for hours that afternoon. The time went by very quickly. This woman had an impact on me that I could not fully comprehend at the time.

By the time Ben picked me up, I was getting extremely sick from the pasta. My stomach pains were bad, and I wanted to throw up. I knew that I should not have eaten that pasta. It was good, but it seemed a little greasy for some reason. We had more appointments that afternoon. I did my best to get through them. My first appointment was with a nurse that fitted me with dilators. I was told about these in advance, but I was surprised that they fit me for them. I sat on the table with my feet in stirrups like at my gynecology appointments. She had a long, clear, rigid, plastic dilator that she inserted into my vagina. It hurt because my lady parts were burnt. She gave me two varied sizes to take home and instructed me to start two weeks after treatment and use them nightly for ten minutes. I asked how long I would have to use the dilators, and she said that it would be good to do it indefinitely or, better yet, to have frequent sex. *Really??* I did not bother to explain my situation to her. She explained that it could shrink down there if I did not. It is a condition called vaginal atrophy, and it is extremely common after pelvic radiation. She also gave me another butt pillow, a squeeze bottle, and a prescription for lidocaine spray. She told me to use the squeeze bottle when I urinated. I was instructed to fill it with tepid water and squirt it on myself while I peed to dilute the urine so it would not sting as much. The lidocaine spray was to be used as needed, right before elimination.

We then went to Dr. Jordan's office. I laid on the table in a fetal position to reduce my stomach cramps. Jackie came in, and I told her I felt sick to my stomach. She handed me a throw-up bag and waited for Dr. Jordan. When he arrived, he asked me what was going on, and I told him that it must have been the pasta I ate. He pressed on my abdomen in a few places and told me to stay away from greasy foods right now. We had a conversation about nutrition. I told him that I was on a vegan diet. He did not object but said that I needed to be careful right now to get enough protein and to stay away from greasy foods and foods that were hard to digest. He admitted that the Keto diet (which is quite different than being vegan) was a valid anti-cancer diet. Let me repeat that. He admitted that the Keto diet was a valid anti-cancer diet. He said that there were studies that backed it up. For real! An oncologist discussing a metabolic approach to cancer! Unheard of! I told him that I liked the Keto diet but did not agree with all the animal fat. There is a trend now toward a Green Keto diet. It's not easy for me to maintain, especially when I don't have the strength to cook for myself.

He looked at my radiation area and said that it looked like it should at this stage. He warned me that things would worsen and prescribed pain meds to take as needed. He also said that my tumor was responding very well to the treatments. He could see that from the scans used during each treatment. Instead of being happy about the tumor shrinking, I wondered what all those CT scans were doing to my body. Lastly, he said that my labs looked good. I could see that my absolute lymphocytes were exceptionally low, and I asked about that. He said that was normal and was from the chemo, but that overall, my white counts were still rather good and that the plan was to start chemo again on Monday. I always analyzed my labs. I looked up a lot online and asked questions about what I did not understand. I told him how worried I was about the next round of chemo, and he said that it would be much better if I would just keep up with my anti-nausea meds and take the pain meds when I needed them. He knew that I was not a fan of pharmaceuticals, so he made a point to tell me that this was not the time for me to try to do this on my own. I thanked him and left with one script for a pain med, another for anxiety, and a salve for burns. I planned to use my salves from the naturopath, and I did not think I needed any meds for anxiety. I wasn't sure about the pain medication. He gave me a low dose of Oxy, and I thought it might still be too strong.

My outpatient surgery never got scheduled for Friday as it should have been, so I had to go to Mayo on a Sunday to get my PICC line put in for my second round of chemo. Not sure who dropped the ball this time, but I have some idea. I went to the hospital building on Sunday morning, and it was a quick procedure. It hurt worse this time because I knew what was coming.

Tony left that evening. I wondered when I would see him again, and I worried about him as usual. I always worried about Tony. I needed to beat this disease and stick around in case he needed me one day. I often imagined that I would be living with him in my old age. I thought we might need to take care of one another.

Some of our friends decided to take care of our dogs for us for the last two weeks of my treatment, so it was back to just the two of us at the casita. It was now hot outside during the day, but I was always cold. It was especially chilly for me in the hospital due to the air conditioning. While most people were dressed in shorts and sandals, I always wore a sweater, shoes, and socks. I also carried my butt pillow with me everywhere I went. I stopped wearing my wigs and found it easier and more comfortable to just wear my scarves. Makeup was also not a priority. I was truly a sight to see, but I could have cared less. I was so listless now that Ben had to drop me off at the door and then go to park the car and meet me in the lobby. When he dropped me at the curb, the Mayo attendants brought me a wheelchair immediately. All they had to do was look at me, and they knew that I needed the chair. They wheeled me into the lobby, where I waited for Ben to take me down to radiation. I never imagined I would be in a wheelchair, but that's how weak I was.

Monday morning, I went to the oncology floor. Dr. Kelson came in while I was there and informed me that I would be getting less of the Mitomycin than my first round. This was due in part to my new weight and my reaction to it in the first round. I had no argument with that. The Five FU had to be the same amount. He said he agreed with Dr. Kumar and would order me the IV combo that included Aloxi and Amend for my anti-nausea meds. This was to be supplemented with Zofran on a timely basis. I should begin tonight before bedtime and every six hours after that. I would also be receiving IV hydration every day for the next four days, immediately after my radiation treatments. Lastly, he prescribed me the steroid pack, and I was to take it starting today for five consecutive days to prevent any possibility of the rash reoccurring. He was on the ball this time. It helps to complain. He also must have gotten word that I had been to the Patient Relations Department three times during my first and second weeks of treatment. I was told each time that someone would call me to discuss my concerns. No one ever did! On my last visit, I asked for another medical oncologist. I did not blame Dr. Kelson. I blamed Dr. Larkin and the department. My complaints were 1) I was told that I had a team that would meet weekly to discuss my status, which was as far as it could be from the truth; 2) Where was Dr. Larkin? I never once saw her after our original consult, and I specifically asked to; 3) Why did it take Dr. Kelson so long to respond to my questions, especially when I complained about chest pain? I did not feel that this was a quality standard of care; 4). Why was I working with a doctor who could not answer any of my questions in a timely fashion? I had to consult with an outside oncologist for the help I needed, and 5). Why isn't anyone from this department contacting me about any of this?

The Mitomycin was given again by "push." My little friend was once again hooked up to me for the next long 96 hours!

That night I was not nauseous, but I was very tired from the new anti-nausea cocktail. I took my Zofran, and it made me feel sick, but I didn't throw up. I ate a little soup and a couple of bites of a grilled cheese sandwich to get something in my stomach and went to bed. I tried to stay as hydrated as possible, but that made me have to urinate more frequently. I started to feel a burning sensation during urination, so I filled my bottle and squirted it while I peed. It helped a little. Bowel movements were now sometimes diarrhea.

I was told that this was from the radiation. They also burned. I used a great deal of the salves and lotions that were prescribed for me. I tried each one for a course to see which worked best for me. It was hard because I had to remove them completely before radiation or burn even worse. It's like wearing baby oil in the sun. My groin area started to blister, and I seriously wondered how I would get through another nine days of radiation. Sleep was my only peace, and I often had vivid dreams. That night I dreamt again about the "bad guy" chasing me.

When I turned back to look, there was no visible figure. I still felt the danger approaching. I ran and felt him gaining on me. At the very last moment, I flew up to the safety of a rooftop. I narrowly escaped. I woke up feeling terrified and afraid of everything I was going through. I also felt a tightness in my chest. I did not know what it was, but I was shaking and weak, and it felt like an elephant was stepping on me. I wondered why the Zantac was not working. I drank some ginger ale, burped, and I felt a bit better. I chalked it up to heartburn, but it really didn't feel like any heartburn that I have ever experienced. It was different.

A few friends came to visit that week. They were friends from the club that also had homes in the valley. I didn't have the heart to tell them not to come, so I did my best to chat with them for a bit. I'm sure they were shocked to see me bald, skinny, pale, and weak. I had always been one of the younger women at the club and so full of energy. *What must I look like now?*

By the end of week five, I was so ready to have my bag removed. I had somehow survived the second round of chemo, thanks to the new meds. Dr. Jordan looked at my burns. He and Jackie must have felt sorry for me. I no longer had the energy to sit up. When he entered the exam room, I was lying on the table in a fetal position and had truly little to say except to answer his questions. He assured me that I would make it through the final week of radiation, and he complimented me on my progress thus far. He also said that it looked like the tumor was now completely gone. He did emphasize that it was important for me to finish my treatments and not give up now because I have come so far already. I cried.

During my final week of radiation treatments, I concentrated on keeping hydrated, and the wonderful crew of techs kept me going with constant praise for my continued strength and endurance. I did get to see John and Eric many more times with a mix of three or four other female techs on occasion. Once or twice, while sitting in the small waiting room, a patient would ring a large brass bell that hung on the wall to signify that they were done with their treatments. All the patients would clap and congratulate them, and sometimes staff would join us. I knew that my time would come soon. I would get to ring the bell on Friday afternoon. I told Ben that I would ring it so hard that I might just knock it off the wall. He challenged me to do just that.

I learned in week six that I could endure more pain than I ever imagined. My private areas were now so raw and blistered that all I could do was to lay in bed with my legs spread apart. It was impossible even to wear panties. I wore Ben's boxer shorts under a dress to my Mayo visits, and in bed, I wore just a nightgown. I had to try to sleep with my legs up and open. When they fell, it would wake me up in tremendous pain. I held off until now with my pain meds, but now I needed them. I took an Oxycodone one night, and I got so sick on it that I phoned the doctor on call and got Tramadol prescribed instead.

Now the pain from eliminating was even worse. It was not unusual for me to scream out with a bowel movement. It felt like I was passing razor blades. This was a common statement relayed by many other Anal Cancer survivors. I had to spray or dab on Lidocaine with every bowel movement first and then bite down on something or hold onto something while defecating. I often let out a scream, and Ben would come running. There was nothing he could do. I just had to get it done. Sometimes when I peed, I would bang my head several times against the side of the open door. It was a ridiculously small bathroom. I found a group of Anal Cancer survivors on Facebook that I consulted with that advised me to purchase a sitz bath, fill it with cool water, and sit in it when I urinated or anytime, I needed some relief. We got one, and I used it a few times, but it was a pain to fill and set up, and it cooled off too quickly for my liking. I missed my bathtub at home, and all we had at the casita was a shower. I looked on Amazon for a small baby blow-up bath that I could place in the bottom of the shower. I found one and ordered it, and it was a great relief. I would sit in it on the bottom of the shower and just let the water spray on my back and into the small pool. It worked perfectly. It felt good while I was in it, but it was difficult for me to get out of, so Ben would have to help me get out. Ben had to help me with everything at this stage. I needed him to cook for me, clean for me, drive me places, and help me get dressed. I wondered when I would be able to do things for myself again. It was strange being so helpless. I felt fortunate that I had help. I imagined that others did not, and I wondered how they got by. In my mind, I wondered if this was Ben's way of acting out an apology for possibly giving me the HPV. I leaned heavily on him, and I knew that it was hard for him to see me like this.

During these last few days, I tended to my wounds and dealt with the pain as best I could. The Facebook survivor's group that I found was an invaluable source. There are approximately 600 members in the group. I then found and joined a second group with over 1,000 members. The members are from all over the world and from all walks of life. We help each other through the treatment and with the various side effects of treatment. It is also great for one's psyche to know that so many others have survived this cancer. The woman who runs one of the groups is a 17-year survivor of stage 4 Anal Cancer. Sometimes it can get depressing to look at posts from others who have it worse, and it can also make me a bit envious of others that caught their cancers earlier than I did. Many of them are stage 1 or 2. There seem to be quite a few members from the UK, and I noticed that their standard of care differs dramatically from that in the US. There are some horror stories that sound like malpractice cases and some others that rave about their teams. Many patients get diagnosed mistakenly with hemorrhoids, just like I did. The majority had bleeding as their first symptom. Some had internal tumors, and others had external tumors, and some even had both. The ones with the external tumors seemed to experience a lot more pain for obvious reasons. It was clear to me that it mattered a great deal where they received treatment. One woman went to a major cancer center and was initially told that she could not have Anal Cancer because it was a gay man's cancer. Are you kidding me? MD Anderson and Memorial Sloan Kettering were said to have a lot more experience than most. Some group members went to their local hospitals, and the care they received was often subpar, but not always. It was just as important to have a dedicated and qualified oncologist as it was to be treated in a superior facility. I knew that to be a fact.

On my last day, we packed up the car and checked out of our casita before treatment. We were anxious to get home and wanted to head back right after our appointments. Ben made me one scrambled egg and a piece of toast for breakfast. It tasted like glue. Ben also helped me to get dressed that morning. We said goodbye to our hosts and thanked them for the accommodations. They wished me a speedy recovery. It was already in the high nineties when we left for the hospital. I wore my blue shirt dress with Ben's boxer shorts underneath. I put on my gold sweater and wore flat, comfortable sandals that day. If I got cold in the waiting rooms or treatment, I could always ask for a pair of those lovely hospital socks with the no-slip rubber on them. I put my wig on and a little lipstick but brought my soft cotton turban to change into for radiation. I did not like wearing the wig in the radiation room.

I had two of the ladies with me for my last radiation treatment, and they were very sweet as usual. I felt sad that I would not get to see John or Eric on my last day. I got on the table and in my position with my bladder filled to 80%. I listened to my R and B music. *Lovely Day* by Bill Withers was playing. As I listened, my thoughts drifted to my first days of radiation and how nervous and fearful I was. I was done after today, and I hoped and prayed that I would never have to go through anything like this again. I also prayed for all the others before me and all those who would come after me not to suffer side effects. I prayed that a cure for this and other cancers would come soon so that this treatment would never again be necessary.

When I was done, the ladies congratulated me for finishing treatment and told me that I was a trooper. I went directly to the bathroom and then to the changing room as I always do. I then returned to the waiting area. There, to my complete surprise, were all my technicians standing in a line. John, Eric, and all the others were waiting for me to ring the bell. I didn't get into my wheelchair like usual. Instead, I walked proudly over to that bell and rang it as loud and proud as I could, and everyone cheered for me. I cried happy tears and thanked them all for always treating me with kindness and respect and for putting up with my sick days and finicky bladder. I noticed that a few patients and techs were also tearing up.

My last stop was Dr. Jordan's office. I was weighed, and my blood pressure was taken as is customary before seeing him. I now weighed in at 125 pounds. I had lost 28 pounds since my diagnosis. If you want to lose weight, I don't recommend this method! My blood pressure was alarmingly low. They took it a couple of times to make sure it was correct. No crossing of legs. Be careful how you hold your arm. Roll up your sleeve. Try again in an upright position. 87/50. It made me think of Ben's dad when he was dying and how his blood pressure dropped. I saw Jackie first, and she took my blood pressure again. No change. She asked me several questions and took notes for Dr. Jordan. I came in with a notepad myself so that I could best manage my recovery at home.

I was afraid of what he would think when he saw my burns. They were bad. My groin was now open wounds that blistered and oozed a yellowish substance. I had both hard and soft blisters in and outside of my lady parts. I had no idea what my anal area looked like, but it felt very raw and both itched and burned at the same time. My hair was completely gone making me look like a twelve-year-old. I got up on the table and into the stirrups, and he looked things over carefully. He was quite pleased and not at all surprised. He wrote me a new prescription for my burns and told me to dab it on as thick as possible at bedtime with a gloved hand. Jackie gave me a box of nitrile gloves. She also gave me a large bag of Aquaphor samples for use during the day. She then told me about a product called Calmoseptine that could be obtained over the counter and would provide a barrier to my skin where necessary. She said that it was a very thick white salve and to put it on with a q-tip. I was instructed to put this around my anus and around my urethra to alleviate the sting from urine or diarrhea.

Dr. Jordan warned me that the radiation burns would get worse before they got better. Today's treatment would hit me a few days later, and yesterday's treatment has not hit me yet. I couldn't imagine things getting worse than this. I thought about burn victims and how much they must suffer. What must it be like to have burns over most of your body? You would have to live on pain pills. Dr. Jordan asked me if I needed a refill on any pain meds and was surprised when I told him that I had barely taken any of them to date. He told me it was not a time to be a hero and to use them as needed. He was not worried about my abusing the pain meds. He knew me pretty well by now. I asked him about my diet and what I should eat to keep my stools soft. I was afraid of constipation from the opioids. He said that anytime I took a pain pill, I should take a Senna laxative. He told me to pick this up at the pharmacy today. Then he thought again and instructed me to take two when I took a pain pill and one every night regardless. He told me that diarrhea was bad, but that constipation would be worse.

Diarrhea was a concern for dehydration, but that could be remedied. Constipation was something that could take time to resolve if I did not act proactively. It would be a balancing act for a while. He warned me that my fatigue would be severe and that it could last for weeks or months. He asked if I had help and then looked at Ben, and he confirmed this would be the case. I asked him when I could expect to be back to normal, and he said I should expect to be golfing again in about three months. I asked about diet and expressed concern about my weight loss, and of course, he said that I could eat whatever I wanted but concentrate on protein. He told me that patients who maintained their weight did better overall than those who lost a lot of weight. He told me not to lose any more weight than I already had. He set up a consultation with a dietician for the next week, Friday afternoon. I would be seeing him again in a week, even though I was done with treatments. I asked him about the dilators and when I should start using them. He said that I could start at any time after about two weeks. I asked him about the trial, and he said that he scheduled the mandatory PET-CT for two months post-treatment.

We would sign me up for the trial at that time because there was no issue with the trial filling up in two months. It would be ongoing for years. He told me that my cancer was no longer detected in the radiation scans and that he was confident that I would have a clear scan for the trial. He was happy that I changed my mind about it and that I was planning to participate. I told him I was very worried about the cancer coming back, and I teared up again. He didn't know what to say. All he could say was how proud he was of my progress, that I was doing great, and that I had come a long way. He said that I should concentrate on my recovery.

"It may look as if the situation is creating the suffering, but ultimately this is not so – your resistance is."

Eckhard Tolle

Chapter 19

Transparency

When I arrived home, I was informed that some of my poker group friends had pitched in and had my house cleaned and my dogs clipped and bathed (well, the little one anyway). Deedee would not go into the van. They hired one of those mobile units. Deedee loves baths but hates trucks. I was gob smacked with the number of cards, flowers, and gifts sitting on my counter. I should send thank you notes or call them all. I should write down who sent a charm or handwritten poem or angel statue with their card because I will forget later. I was too tired just thinking about all of it. I hoped they would forgive me. Of course, Ben and I thanked the girls who watched and bathed my dogs and had my house cleaned. I had the president of our women's golf association send a letter to our members from me. Since she let them know when I was going into treatment, it was only right that I now should update them on my status. This is what I sent out:

Dear Friends and PLWGA Members,

As I stare out my window at my beautiful view with serene azure skies, I hear the sounds of spring with birds chirping in their varied songs. My dogs are prancing around the yard just waiting for something to bark at, and Ben is laughing at sports highlights on TV. It all makes me feel grateful for what I have.

Many of you have been asking how I am doing, so I want to update you all. I have completed my treatments at Mayo with much help from my family and good friends. I am now back home for my recovery. It was much harder than I anticipated. My doctors are proud of me for finishing this very aggressive protocol. I still have a long way to go but hope to be back up and around by late summer in some golfing capacity. That is my goal, anyway. I will be traveling back to Mayo for follow-ups in the next couple of weeks, and since the treatments keep working even after they are completed, no scans will be done for several weeks. I am also considering a clinical trial for an immunotherapy drug which will be administered monthly for the next six months if I am chosen. This helps my body to fight any stubborn cells that may remain. It is, without a doubt, still a lot of trips to the doctor, but I am thrilled to be HOME.

I can't tell you how much I have appreciated all your cards, gifts, visits, flowers, offers of assistance, meals, prayers, and words of encouragement. My home is filled with your thoughtfulness. Your greetings, etc... have kept me hopeful on days when I have felt really low. Many of you commented on how strong I am and that I am a fighter, but I often feel just very weak and unsure of how to handle all these symptoms and side effects. I am overanxious to get back to normal although I think I may never be that same person again.

Thank you again for thinking of me during this challenging time in my life. I am most grateful for all your friendships. Looking forward to getting stronger and seeing all of you again at the club or around town. It is a beautiful time of the year.

Love,
Bonnie

I was living in a complete sea of confusion. I was a bit overwhelmed with everything. Part of this could be what they call "chemo brain." I knew that I needed to concentrate on my supplements again, start juicing and begin my high-dose vitamin IV protocol, but I was too weak to put my pills together and too sick to take them. I was too tired to bathe or get dressed, so I only did what I had to. I could do no more than the basics right now. I had to eat. I had to manage my pain. I had to balance my bowels. I concentrated on my basic physical health only. It was a lot of headbanging into the side of my bathroom door. It was calling out for help when I got dizzy and too weak to get out of the bathtub or shower. It was a lot of calling Ben and reminding him about my meds.

I wished I had my daughter to set up a schedule for Ben. He did his best, but we had no real plan. We just winged it. On day three, I did not have a bowel movement. It was concerning. I couldn't remember if I even had one on day two. I took an extra Senna. It is a natural laxative and takes time to work. It was not working. On day four, I started feeling sick. I mean, really sick. I should have started taking the Senna sooner, just like with the anti-nausea meds. The nurse warned me about constipation with my pain meds. I just forgot to take them. I was nauseous. My stomach hurt. My back hurt. I felt more lethargic than ever. I couldn't eat. I was not drinking enough. I wondered what was causing my constipation. I looked up the causes, and I had almost all of them. I was dehydrated as I had gotten lax about drinking enough water. I was taking pain meds (opioids). I had a narrowed rectum due to the fissures and inflammation from radiation. I had additional radiation damage to the nerves in my rectum (autonomic neuropathy). My pelvic muscles no longer relaxed and contracted correctly (dyssynergia). I had weakened pelvic muscles. I was getting little to no physical activity. I wasn't eating enough fiber right now, and I was depressed. It was as though I checked off every box under the causes for constipation. I finally got so sick that I had to call the doctor. He told me to get a stronger laxative and take it at bedtime. That day was horrible. I had bad constipation only two other times in my life after the birth of my children. This was ten times worse. Every time I strained even just a little, I would just have gas, bleed, or pass a little mucus. Sorry if this is gross. I felt so bloated. I was getting a little diarrhea at the same time, but I could not pass the rest of the stool. I felt bloated in my chest as well. I drank ginger ale and felt a little better after I burped. Ben took a late-night trip to the CVS and purchased fast-acting Dulcolax. I took it as directed and tried my best to sleep without a pain pill that night. I tossed, turned, and had a horrible night. Early the next morning, I experienced explosive bloody diarrhea. It came with waves of painful cramping. I was shaking and sweating. I went from one extreme to the next. Now what? It was bad, but it was better than constipation.

I made it a point to drink at least four large glasses of water each day, and I decided I would not take any more pain pills. Instead, I depended on my lidocaine to relieve myself, and I took Azo to dilute my urine. I would also continue to bang my head on the corner of the bathroom door. It's just what I did when it hurt. Ben caught me doing it one time and said, "What the hell are you doing?" I told him that it helped me while I passed my razor blades!

Friends came to visit. They brought casseroles, cookies, and gifts. Sadly, most of the food was never eaten. Someone planted some beautiful flowers in a large pot near the front of my house. I asked a few of the ladies that I thought might have planted them, but no one fessed up. Instead, they offered to help with whatever Ben, or I needed. I needed nothing, but I needed everything. Some stopped by and sat with me. They told me that I looked good and was the bravest person they knew, but they could not mean it. I looked like shit. I couldn't stand looking at myself in the mirror. My muscles had atrophied. I was bald. I had dark circles under my eyes. My skin was darkened in patches where my rash was. I was burned and peeling where the radiation did its thing. My eyes were lifeless, and my smile had turned to an almost constant frown. I now had frown lines, and bags, which I worried would be permanent. I was a mere shadow of the woman I once was. I remember one of our friends saying, "you look ..." and she hesitated and then said, "comfortable." She couldn't lie. It was the best compliment she could produce.

Every spring, our club has a tournament that they call "Monster Day." It is a four-person scramble. I usually play with the same ladies, and we have come in first place for the lady's division for the last two years. Our team leader, Janine, texted me and asked me if I would be up for company for a couple of minutes as our group (with one new player taking my place) made the turn from hole nine to hole ten. We live right off hole nine. I reluctantly agreed to the visit even though I was not feeling anywhere near up to it. She told me that she would warn me when they were on hole eight. That day, Ben told me that groups were stopping by and tying balloons to my front gate. By the time I got myself up to look outside my front door, several balloons were out there. I was surprised and humbled. My group texted me, and I got ready. With Ben's help, I put on a pair of jeans, but they were so loose that they fell off. I found a pair of leggings that still fit, and I threw on a t-shirt. I wore my wig and even put on a little makeup.

I looked at myself one last time in the mirror and hated what I saw. I met them out front, knowing they would be on a tight schedule to get to the next hole. They were all wearing the same purple t-shirts that had a screen-printed picture of me in my long pink curly wig (the one I tried on at the Wig Shop) and sent to her by text a few weeks ago.) It read "Bonnie's Monsters" underneath and the date. Janine handed me a bag while the other ladies tied more balloons to my gate. I was asked to put my shirt on so they could take a picture. I didn't really want a picture, but how could I refuse. Ben snapped a photo of the five of us in our matching shirts with the balloons behind us. It was a nice gesture that I will never forget. Before they left, they said that Margaret (another friend who sometimes sits for my dogs) dedicated the tournament to me.

She made the announcement that morning to the whole club. It was very touching, and I teared up thinking about it. I missed my old life even though I was never this popular prior to my cancer diagnosis.

That afternoon I got a call from Paul Cassidy. He oversaw Patient Relations at the Mayo Clinic. They were finally returning my call! He started the conversation by saying that he was extremely sorry for the delay. He offered no excuse for why it took so long. I would have thought that he could have produced a lie, but he did not even try. I made sure he knew that I had gone to his office a total of three times. He knew it. He just kept saying that he had no excuse and that he was deeply sorry. I told him how unhappy I was with the Medical Oncology Department and Dr. Larkin (ghost). He asked me if I still wanted to change oncologists. I told him that I had to contact an outside oncologist during my treatment because I could not get answers from Dr. Larkin or Dr. Kelson. I sarcastically reminded him that I was now done with treatment. I don't think he even knew that.

Mr. Cassidy said that he could give my file to a Dr. Li. Dr. Li was their most senior medical oncologist on staff at Mayo, and he felt that I would find him very professionally qualified. I told him I would be willing to meet with him for my future aftercare. It sounded like Dr. Kelson was fired, or he may have quit. I imagined that if I was that dissatisfied with him, others were as well, and if I were him and had to work under Dr. Larkin, I would want to find a better situation. I also said that I was disappointed in the care that I received from Medical Oncology as a whole and that I was not the only patient to express those concerns. He said that he understood completely and again apologized. The last thing I said was that I hoped that the department would learn something and set better care standards. I said that if the entire department had that reputation, then it likely came from the top. He agreed. I voiced some of the concerns that I and others experienced, such as long wait times for chemo, missed deadlines, poor communication, inexperienced and/or missing nurses and physicians, and worst of all, misdiagnoses. Where was this part of my so-called "team?" I praised the radiation department from Dr. Jordan on down to the nurses and technicians. I wondered how two departments could be so different.

On Friday, Ben and I drove to Mayo for a two-week post-treatment follow-up. The drive went by quickly. It was so routine to us now.

I weighed in at 118 pounds. I had lost another seven pounds in just the last week alone. This was genuinely concerning to me. When I looked at myself in the mirror now, I could see my rib bones. I looked anorexic. Jackie had a worried look on her face. I was so listless. I was slumped down on the bench next to Ben when she came in. She asked me how I was doing, and I told her my concerns. I was weak all the time. I couldn't do anything for myself. The only thing I managed to do alone was go back and forth to the toilet when I needed to. Mostly I stayed in bed or in the recliner. I know this sounds strange, but I missed walking my dogs. I missed cooking and even cleaning my house.

I told her that I was still having issues with my bowel movements. They were very loose, and I could not always make it to the bathroom. I could hold my urine in but not my stools. I asked her if this would get better. She wrote that question down for the doctor. So far, I did not have to wear pads, but I did not go anywhere. I was just making it to the bathroom from my bed. Luckily, I had my bowel movements in the morning. She asked me how many I was having a day, and I told her at least three or four, but they were all in the early part of the day. It still hurt badly to go, even though it was mostly diarrhea. Was that normal? She kept taking notes. I was also having a tough time eating. I felt full all the time. I was getting stomach aches after I ate. It felt to me like I was not digesting certain foods. She took more notes to go over with Dr. Jordan. He came in and looked things over. He was pleased again with my progress on my burns. He saw signs that they were beginning to heal in certain areas. I thought to myself, that's just the outside.

What about my insides? He told me that the fatigue was normal and that it would take time to get back to my old self. He said that the pain with my stools was normal and to use the lidocaine. He was not sure about the stomach issues. He said that the dietician would address those issues with me. He thought that I could potentially control this with my diet. I wanted more answers, but there were none to be had. He said I lost muscle tone, so I will have little to no notice when moving my bowels. This, he believed, would get better, and if it did not, there were exercises that I could do to improve my muscle tone. It's Kegel exercises where you squeeze your bottom and hold it for a minute or two and then let go. I told him that I was exercising in bed as much as possible. He said that was great. I had hand weights and did leg lifts every day. He told me to try and walk around as much as possible. Ha! That was a bit humorous.

As for the digestion issues, he thought those could be related to the chemo. He said that Dr. Li could better address those issues on my next appointment or call him before if things did not improve. He said that he would not see me again until June 29. That was the date of my PET/CT scan. On that day, I would get full labs and the scans in the morning and meet with Dr. Jordan and then with the new medical oncologist, Dr. Li, in the afternoon. I was looking forward to meeting him. I was looking forward to feeling better by this next appointment.

I then met with the dietician. I thought she looked young. I sat down, expecting that she would understand the effects of chemo on my GI tract and give me solutions to my digestion issues, stomach cramps, and diarrhea. Instead, she showed me plastic pieces of lean protein meats, fish, and vegetables, and showed me a wide variety of sugary protein drinks such as Ensure. She did not have answers to any of my questions. Instead, she diverted to her plastic pieces and told me to keep my weight up. Well, duh! If I could eat, things would be much easier. She gave me a goody bag, and I left. It was a complete waste of my time.

It was beautiful outside, and all I could do was watch the sun come up and go down. I could listen to the birds gleefully chirping at our feeders. I could also hear golfers on the tee box. Ben was now back to a full schedule of golf. That means for him a five-day schedule. I was happy for him. He needed to get away. I was alone for several days a week and for several hours a day, and this was a pivotal time for me. I used this time to reflect on my life. I cried a lot. I had so much anxiety built up in me, and sometimes I just needed to let it all out. I started a journal. It was mostly just my feelings, thoughts, and fears. I knew that I had to make a change. I had to stop living in fear and feeling sorry for myself, but I felt like a mere shadow of my old self.

I decided to try to walk the dogs one day when Ben was golfing. It took most of my energy to get dressed and put the harnesses on the dogs. I looked like hell. I had my turban on and long pants and a long-sleeved shirt. It was 80 degrees outside, but I could not chance a sunburn, and my head would get chilly if there was a breeze. The dogs were surprisingly patient with me. Pita did not pull like he normally did. Maybe they understood more than I gave them credit for? I got just a few yards down the street, and fatigue set in. I was determined to fight through it. I needed a rest, so I sat down on the sidewalk. The dogs were incredibly good. They seemed concerned and waited for me. A neighbor that knew us well drove by and saw me. He was obviously concerned and pulled the car over to ask if I was okay. I told him that I was fine and just needed a rest. He asked if he could drive me somewhere or walk the dogs for me, and I told him that I wanted to try and do it myself. He said okay and drove very slowly away. I got up after a bit and continued to the trail. As I neared the entrance to the trail, I saw my neighbor drive by again. He was kindly checking up on me.

I started off on the trail and quickly realized that I had bitten off more than I could chew. The dogs peed and pooped. I bent over to bag Deedee's poop, and I got dizzy trying to get back up. I lost my balance and fell over. I quickly looked around to see if anyone saw me. I was happy no one was around. I sat there with the poop bag, trying to hold both leashes. It smelled so bad. I let go of the leashes to tie up the bag. The dogs were fantastic. They stayed right by my side. I got the leashes back in hand and rested until I was ready to go again. Getting up was quite another challenge on the rocky uphill grade, but I did it! I was proud of myself. It was now finally all downhill. I got to the end of the trail and crossed over to the sidewalk again. I needed another rest, so I sat down again. This time Ben came speeding down the street in our golf cart yelling at me. He told me that he was planning to walk the dogs as soon as he got home. I told him that I knew that but that I wanted to try it. He seemed a little angry with me.

He said, "What if the dogs pulled you down?"

I told him that they were good, and they did not pull me at all. I left out the part where I fell over. We took the ride home in the golf cart, mostly because the dogs love the golf cart so much. I told Ben about the neighbor stopping, and he said that the neighbor called him. I hoped he did not end his golf round early because of me, and he said he was on the last hole anyway. Well, I thought to myself, I had better let him know next time I planned such a big outing!

About a month after treatment ended, I thought I was finally getting a little stronger, and then I started to have that odd chest pressure. It was worse after I ate, and I was eating extraordinarily little. I now did not want to eat at all. I was also still having issues with my bowels. I tried to keep a log of what foods caused me digestion issues. It was exceedingly difficult. I decided to eliminate dairy from my diet. Many people told me that dairy could be hard to digest. I had already eliminated most other fats and sugar. I knew that I could not eat fatty meats, fried foods, or fresh vegetables. I knew this because the grill at the club prepared a large meal for me after one of Ben's golf events, and I ate about a quarter of it. It was truly kind of them, and it tasted delicious. They told me that they were only happy to prepare meals for me at any time. It was some sort of a pot roast with crispy baby red potatoes and carrots. After a couple of hours, I got really sick. After that I would never eat from the grill. I could eat cooked potatoes and carrots at home without issue, so I figured it must have been the meat or the oil that they used to fry the potatoes in. I simply could not digest food like I used to. I also tried to eat salads and got sick from those. I tried to eat tiny pieces of steak one night, and that did not go over well. I tried chicken salad and tuna salad without success. I then took on a very bland diet. Some of the items I could eat successfully were oatmeal, baked pears or apples, mashed potatoes, cooked carrots, bananas, scrambled eggs, and toast.

I didn't understand why I had this pain in my chest. It did not seem like heartburn, but they say chest pain and heartburn can be difficult to differentiate. I tried to burp by drinking carbonated water, but I could not. It seemed like I was getting bloated. It was as if food was getting stuck in my esophagus. This side effect started to set me back, and I wanted to figure out why this was affecting me. I got on my blogs and asked other survivors if they had these symptoms, and most did not, or they had different symptoms. I also made an appointment with my primary care physician Dr. Singh. When the nurse took my blood pressure, it was 75/55! She was concerned and took it again. Not much better. I looked horrible. Dr. Singh asked me how I was doing, and I cried. I cried a lot these days. I told him that I felt as though an elephant was standing on my chest. I told him that I could not eat and felt I was not digesting my foods properly. I asked him if I was dying. Singh said that this was my GI tract. He said that the chemotherapy kills all my fast-growing cells, most of which are in my GI tract. He also felt that I could have some pancreatic insufficiency. I asked about pancreatic enzymes, and he said that those were fine to take short term, but I should not take them long-term or my body would not learn to produce its own enzymes again. He said that my system was like that of a baby now. Everything that died off needed to come back.

I was angry that my oncologists did not warn me about this. It was like mouth sores, but they were in my esophagus and further down my GI tract as well. Dr. Singh gave me a solution of lidocaine that I was told to swallow. Really? I'm supposed to swallow lidocaine. It's a small amount, and it was mixed with something to coat my esophagus. I held on to the prescription. He also gave me a prescription for an anti-anxiety med and a steroid for I don't know what. He also told me to buy psyllium powder to gel up my stools. I needed to put a tablespoon of this in my water daily. He also told me to get more protein in my diet. I should try lentils and drink three or four good-quality protein drinks daily. His instructions were like a sea of confusion. I could not comprehend most of what he was telling me, and I was overwhelmed. I took notes, but then I lost them. He did not understand that when I felt the chest pressure, I could not eat, could not drink, and I could not take pills. I left there feeling quite helpless.

I reached out to Jackie on the portal, and Dr. Jordan called me back the next morning. He said that he would refer me to their GI department for a consult. I was scheduled to see Dr. Snyder in five days. I remembered how CTCA had a GI doctor on my team, and now I knew why that was. That night I ended up in the Emergency room at Yavapai Regional. I was listless, my heart was pounding, and the elephant was not letting up. I was immediately put into a wheelchair because I was too weak to walk. The intake nurse asked Ben what was wrong, and as soon as he said chest pain, we were wheeled into a room, my shirt was opened, and cold, clammy stickers were attached to my chest and ribcage.

The EKG was normal, so I was sent back to the waiting room. There we sat for what seemed like forever. My shaking listless body was just falling to one side in that super uncomfortable ER wheelchair. Ben was getting angry at how long it took to see a doctor. Finally, we got a room, where they hooked me up to monitors and gave me a warm blanket. The warm blankets were the best. It seemed like my blood pressure was taken every 15 minutes or so. It was registering 76/55 when the doctor finally came in and asked me what was going on. I filled him in on my recent treatments, and he looked concerned. I told him that I was having a hard time eating and drinking, and he told his nurse to put me on an IV for hydration. I explained the pain in my chest, and he ordered a solution that I was to drink. It was awful. It was the lidocaine solution that Dr. Singh said would coat my esophagus. It didn't do much. They also gave me something for anxiety, and that's when I finally felt a little better. It was a five-hour ordeal. I don't think you can ever go to the ER and get home in less than five hours. I was so tired when we finally got home. Pita and Deedee were very confused. They didn't understand why we left so suddenly and then came home in the middle of the night.

The next morning, I woke up, and the pain was back. It did not last all day. Thank God. It came and went. Something was very wrong. My body was trying to tell me something, and I didn't know what. I did not know how to help myself, and the doctors did not know how to help me either. Was I supposed to live on Lorazepam, take steroids, and drink Lidocaine every day? This seemed wrong to me. I called Dr. Rubin's office. I begged to get a phone consultation with him, and they fit me in on a cancellation. I told him that I was too sick to take any of my supplements. I explained the chest pains I was having and that my EKG had been normal at the ER. I told him about my difficulties eating and how much weight I had lost, He seemed really concerned. He told me to go out and buy a protein drink called Orgain. It was vegan and would provide me with much-needed calories, vitamins, and protein. I was supposed to drink four to five of these per day. He advised a few supplements to help my GI tract to heal. These came in liquid and powder to mix into my water, so I would not have to take pills. He advised a few types of foods to add to my diet and told me to keep hydrated with warm ginger and peppermint teas and water. He also suggested Aloe for my stomach. I did not know if I could stomach that right now. Lastly, he told me to get an IV of amino acids. He thought that I might be able to find this in Prescott. Again, I was swimming in a sea of confusion. I could not take all the meds that Dr. Singh wanted me to take while taking Dr. Rubin's whole protocol, and what about the after-treatment protocol that Dr. Zander had suggested. I had purchased all that months ago with a plan to start taking them right after treatment ended. I still needed to work on my immune system because I did not want this cancer to return. I desperately did not want that!

"Hope is being able to see the light in spite of the darkness."

Desmond Tutu

Chapter 20

Depression

I know that I cannot accurately describe the pain I was feeling but suffice to say that this was the lowest point in my life thus far. I felt as though my heart was being crushed. All the doctors said that I was experiencing a type of heartburn that was caused by chemotherapy. Oh, I did not doubt that what I was going through was caused by the chemo drugs, but did I think it was heartburn? Hell no! I had experienced heartburn before, and this was nothing of the sort. Did it feel like open sores in my esophagus? Not really. I guess it could be because I didn't know what that felt like. I started looking up the side effects of the Five FU and Mitomycin. Well, I found out that it CAN affect your heart and that patients die from heart complications from these meds. What the hell? A woman I communicated with on the Anal Cancer group told me that her oncologist said that the drugs literally eat away at your heart muscle. Why didn't my doctors warn me about this? Why was my EKG normal then?

Ben drove me to the Mayo Clinic again for my consult with the GI doctor. I liked her a lot. She was a fellow working under Dr. Jiminez, and I met with both of them. They asked me many questions and finally decided that I should have an upper endoscopy and be put on an antacid. Even though I was already taking Zantac, Dr. Snyder wanted me to start on Prilosec immediately. It would take about five days to begin working. They wanted to see if it would make a difference. Dr. Jimenez would do my endoscopy next week. I was also given a strict diet to follow. It was to avoid fried foods, spicy foods, processed foods, and dairy, which I was already doing. Lastly, Dr. Snyder suggested I avoid carbonated beverages as they can make the situation worse. I did not know that. I would need to give up my LaCroix water. Boo. Another protocol to follow by yet another doctor. It's no wonder I had anxiety.

I kept losing weight. I looked at myself in the mirror and felt like a prisoner of war. That was exactly how I looked. My rib cage showed, my whole backbone was visible, my stomach was inverted, and my beautiful bottom was now just sagging wrinkles. My eyes were sunken in. Heavy lines could now be seen at the sides of my mouth and under my jaw. I thought these might be from grimacing. I weighed in at a pathetic 107 pounds. That is down from 152 pre-diagnosis. I knew that I could not lose any more weight. I had been advised to track my calories, so I started a journal on my phone. Each day, I would attempt to eat 1200 calories. Here is an example of one of the days in my journal:

Breakfast
Oatmeal with berries 300
Honey 30
Total breakfast 330
Lunch
Orgain. 220
Banana 100
Juice 30
Total lunch 350
Dinner
Fried rice with egg 280
Mashed potato 160
Chicken 60
Total Dinner 500
Total Tuesday 1180

Well, I soon found out that I could not even get close to my goals. For breakfast, Ben would make me a big bowl of oatmeal with cut up berries or bananas and cinnamon. I forced myself to eat two or three tablespoons. Before he went to golf, he would make me a baked pear with cinnamon. I usually ate all of that over a period of about an hour. I then read, researched, or wrote in my journal. I was getting very depressed, but I did not know it until much later. It began with the pain in my chest, and then the anxiety set in, followed by a fear of dying a painful death. It is important to distinguish that my fear was not of dying but of dying a slow and painful death. I thought about my future, and it frightened me beyond measure. I thought about dying A LOT. The anxiety was deep and made the pain in my chest worse. I could feel the pain and anxiety at the same time. They were feeding off one another like two enemies attacking me at the same time. In the next few weeks, Ben would take me three more times to the ER! Pain and Anxiety were winning this battle. I let them take me down. I was too weak to fight back.

On my second trip to the ER, we just said, "chest pains" and got right in. Again, the EKG was normal. I began to think that the doctors were right, and this was just a bad case of heartburn or something to do with my stomach not closing properly. However, I was not like other Anal Cancer patients. Most of them had bad mouth sores during chemotherapy (mine were quite mild), complained about burns, or had issues with neuropathy. My burns were bad, but they were nothing compared to this feeling in my chest. Why was I the only one with this side effect? Maybe I was one of the lucky ones who had heart failure that did not kill them. They hydrated me, gave me the lidocaine cocktail, an antacid, an anti-anxiety drug, and sent me home. Maybe I should be doing all these things at home. Easier said than done. I decided that I would take more of the Lorazepam since that was the one thing that seemed to help a little. I started to take a half tablet during the day plus my usual full tablet at night. I felt very discouraged that I could not get through this without medication, and I felt that I was only masking the problem and not finding the underlying cause of why this was happening to me.

We went again to Mayo for my Upper Endoscopy. I was hopeful that I would finally get some answers. We went to the other location in Scottsdale for my procedure. The whole floor was dedicated to gastrointestinal procedures. It was amazingly large and efficient. I came in on an empty stomach as instructed. That was not difficult. I was told that I would be given anesthesia for this procedure and that I would not feel a thing. Dr. Jiminez would be going down my throat with a camera and looking at my throat, esophagus, and stomach for any abnormalities. When I got the anesthesia, I was in heaven. I understood completely how people got hooked on pain meds. I then had the best sleep I had in months. It was over all too quickly. The next day the doctor called with my results and said that he did not see anything concerning. I had a small hiatal hernia that they did not seem concerned with. I was negative for Celiac Disease. There was no inflammation noted, and the biopsies and bacterial cultures from my small bowel were normal as well.

I was right. This was not from sores in my esophagus. She told me that the next test would determine if my stomach was closing all the way after I ate my food. This flap is like a muscle that could have been damaged, and if it did not close properly, I could get heartburn. It is called an Esophageal Manometry[xxiv] test, and it measures the function of the lower esophageal sphincter (the valve that prevents reflux, or backward flow, of gastric acid into the esophagus) and the muscles of the esophagus. The test would consist of a nurse putting a tube down my throat and a monitor on me that would record how my food traveled down my esophagus and into my stomach and if that flap was working. The only way to know this was for me to have this tube in me for a few days while the monitor recorded the findings.

I set up the test, but the more I researched it, the more I didn't like the idea of having it done. I heard that it was very painful, could cause an infection, and that it would be hard to eat and sleep with that tube down my throat. It was put in through my nostril. That sounded awful to me. I was hoping that the antacid would work. If it did, then I would cancel the manometry test. I had huge doubts about all of this. It just did not feel like I had heartburn or acid reflux, but I could be wrong, and I needed to find the underlying cause of this.

Every morning I woke up hoping I would get past this side effect. I hoped that it was just something caused by the chemo drugs and that whatever was damaged would repair itself with time. Instead, it was getting worse and not better, and I was getting increasingly anxious about it. It started to affect my breathing. I began to think it was some type of panic attack. Ben did not know what to do for me. He insisted that I go to the ER when he could not help me. On my third trip, the EKG (negative again) was done right away as usual, but we waited four hours to get called in. I was again very weak, shaking, dehydrated, and in pain. I was now 106 pounds and looked anorexic. When I finally got called in, there was no bed. They asked me if I minded being treated in the hallway just until a room became available. I never did get the room. I was desperate for help, and I did not want to wait any longer. I was treated much the same way as I was in the past, but this time, I got a doctor who seemed more concerned about my heart. He hooked me up to the EKG again, did a chest X-ray, and ordered a couple of extra blood tests. He asked me a lot about the chemotherapy drugs I took, and I saw him researching something on the computer. I wish I remembered his name, but I do not. He was kind to take those extra steps to try and diagnose me. It was obvious that this was not heartburn to him. He said that the Five FU could be affecting my heart in a way that would not show up on an EKG. The lady in my Anal Cancer group was right. These drugs were probably eating away at my heart muscles. I told him that the only thing that really helped me was the hydration and the anti-anxiety meds. He had me hydrated and gave me some IV Lorazepam which helped me a great deal. The doctor said that he ruled one thing out but that he was not an expert on those drugs. He suggested that I contact my oncologists and ask for a referral to a cardiologist for further testing, just in case. Why was this the first doctor to bring up cardiac issues with me when I told them for weeks now that it feels like something is wrong with my heart?

The next day, I reached out to Dr. Li at Mayo via the portal. He said that he saw nothing in my labs to indicate any issues with my heart but that he would check them again on the 29th when I came in for my scans. I did not have the strength to argue with him. He said that I should follow up with the test that Dr. Snyder suggested and take my Prilosec. I had stopped taking it because I did not think it was working. Dr. Li got a little ticked off when I mentioned that I started to take Ranitidine (milder than Prilosec) instead. He sternly told me to take the Prilosec two times a day as directed. To me, that was too much. When you read the label, it says not to take the max dose for more than ten days, and it lists a slew of side effects. Again, I did not argue with him. I switched back to the Prilosec, even though I knew it was not helping with my chest pain. I had not even met him yet, and already I didn't care for Dr. Li.

So, now I'm back on the maximum dose of Prilosec two times a day, a Lorazepam after breakfast, and another at bedtime. The only time I am not in pain is when I nap in the afternoon from the Lorazepam and when I sleep at night, thanks again to the Lorazepam. I won't even go into the side effects of the long-term use of anti-anxiety meds!

Ben was getting desperate for answers too. He would come home from golf and find me crying in the recliner on most days. He felt frustrated at not being able to help me. He golfed with an ER doctor one day and asked him what he could do for me. He came to visit me that afternoon after golf and spent a lot of time asking me questions about my symptoms and history. He told me that I should be taking the max dose of Prilosec and not worry about the side effects. He said that the drug works well and should help with my pain. It was extraordinarily nice of him to see me, but he was just like the others and dismissed my pain as heartburn.

It was difficult for me to cook for myself. Ben made sure that I always had something easy to microwave or snack on before he left. I did my best to keep my caloric intake up, but I must admit that I was worried that I might need a feeding tube. A friend of mine is a personal trainer and wellness coach with a master's degree in nutrition I called her for help. We discussed how I could get the calories I needed through healthy fats. I explained that I could not digest certain foods. She made notes, did some research, and got back to me with some ideas for different foods. She suggested a daily smoothie and provided me with recipes. She likes the Orgain drinks that I was already drinking every day. I told her that I was supposed to be drinking four of them per day but that I currently only drank one or two. She seemed genuinely concerned and wanted to help me. She explained that a feeding tube should be my very last resort. I began adding avocados to my diet and several other good fats. This did not go over very well. I got extremely sick from the avocados. I did not understand that at all. I started to drink bone broth which helped a lot. I was grateful for her guidance.

My friend Fran was concerned for me and decided to make a trip to see me from Seattle. She is a chef and brought some homemade soups with her including a huge pot of miso broth. She made a couple of other dishes and portioned them into smaller containers for my freezer. I think she was quite surprised at how weak and feeble I was and how little I could eat. I confided to her that I no longer wanted to live like this anymore and that if it went on like this much longer that I would be looking for a way out. She did not know what to say. I later regretted putting this much weight on her. Of course, she told me to eat and that I would get a little stronger every day, but I did not believe any of it. I was way behind schedule. Other survivors were back to work after a month, and here I was two months out and couldn't even take a shower or eat without help. I was much worse today than I was the days immediately after treatment. Those were supposed to be my worst days, according to my doctors and other survivors.

I finally found an infusion center across from the hospital where I could obtain the amino acids that Dr. Rubin suggested. These were supposed to help with issues such as malabsorption and maldigestion. I remember the IV was very expensive and not covered by my insurance. I felt very fortunate that I could afford this. They also had to get it directly from the hospital. I was very weak the day I had it done and did not feel better immediately after like I had hoped. I probably should have done more than one infusion, but it was a difficult outing for me to undertake without assistance.

I also had a friend suggest acupuncture to me. I was willing to try anything. I made an appointment with Jean Painter, DpOM, CH, Ac., L.Ac.[xxv] Please don't ask me what all that stands for, but she had been voted the best acupuncturist in Prescott for seven years running. It was worth a try. I got a ride from Ben, and while waiting in her office, I noticed a book with letters and comments from satisfied patients. Most of her patients came in with back pain, allergies, or various other ailments. They all praised her treatments. I had never had acupuncture before, so I did not know what to expect. Jean was not very chatty. She was all business and often looked like she was in a bad mood, but that was just her demeanor. She was confident in her abilities to help me with my symptoms. She asked me about my symptoms and treated me for heartburn and anxiety. I laid in a recliner in a wonderfully comfortable room that was decorated with Chinese art and furniture. She had been trained there. She took my blood pressure before we started and seemed concerned. I told her that it was always low. She wiped a few spots on my calves and arms and wrists with alcohol and tapped very thin needles into those areas. They did not hurt, and they did not seem to go very deep. She started to tap one into the top of my head, and I said, wait and took off my wig first. She put a blanket on me, turned the lights down, and turned on some relaxing music which consisted of flutes and a rainstorm. I felt very relaxed and fell asleep after a few minutes. When she entered the room again, she suggested that I come three times per week if I could, and I agreed. I liked how easily I fell asleep, and sleep was getting harder and harder for me. I asked her if it was okay that I slept, and she said that it was optimal. Her sessions cost me 55 dollars each and were not covered by my insurance.

Word must have gotten out at the club that I was experiencing a challenging recovery. I got calls and texts often offering help with rides to appointments. Friends would often call on their way to the grocery store to ask if they could pick anything up for me. I started to take them up on their offers. Joy often drove me to my acupuncture appointments. She said it was perfect because she could do a little shopping at Sprouts while I was being treated. I often had her pick up some fruit or vegetables for me while she was there. On one occasion, I was terribly ill when she brought me in, and she waited for me.

Jean was worried about me too, especially after taking my blood pressure. She asked me when I had eaten anything last, and I told her that I just felt like my chest was being crushed inside a vice, and I wasn't hungry. I showed her my protein drink and took a few sips of it. She went to her kitchen and brought out a plate of gluten free crackers and organic sheep's milk cheese. I sat in a chair and ate what she brought me. After I felt a little better, she gave me my treatment. I did not sleep this time, but I did relax a little. She spent at least two hours with me, and Joy waited for me the whole time. I felt like I was imposing on them, but I could not walk without assistance. I was dizzy and extremely weak.

I started getting homemade soups and casseroles delivered to my house by concerned friends and neighbors. They heard that I was having a difficult time eating. I explained how everything made me sick, so they made dishes for me with simple, easily digestible ingredients. I appreciated these gestures, and I felt good about eating something healthier than the boxed and canned soups that Ben prepared.

These were very dark days for me. I often thought about ending my life. I was tired of being in pain. I was tired of being a burden. I woke up in pain and went to bed in pain. It was now with me 24/7. This pain made my world exceedingly small. My body used to be an instrument that I controlled with my mind. It could no longer act on my will, at least not in any reliable manner. If I desired a glass of water, I might not be able to get it for myself. If my phone was ringing in another room, I just listened until it stopped. If my dogs barked to go outside, I often could not even travel to the next room to open the door for them. My bedroom or my recliner was where I spent both days and nights.

June 29th was coming up, and I would be getting my labs and 2-month scans to determine my eligibility for the Opdivo trial. I would see both Dr. Jordan and Dr. Li in the afternoon. I had so many questions to ask them, and I hoped they could help me find the underlying causes to my issues.

My friend Fran must have told some of our other friends about my feelings of not wanting to live, so I received phone calls from many of them. They were concerned and tried to cheer me up. Fran planned a 60th birthday celebration for all of us Notre Dame girls. Everyone was going to meet up in Prescott to celebrate. I think they were hoping that they could give me something to look forward to.

My friend Kitty from Sedona called me and talked to me about a man named Steve. She knew about Steve from another friend of hers that owns a Crystal Shop in Sedona. Steve is what is known as a Remote Healer. Kitty asked me if I was familiar with Joe Dispenza,[xxvi] and I was not. She explained that he was an Energy Healer and that many such healers could potentially help me with some of my issues. She told me to listen to some YouTube videos from Joe Dispenza and call this Steve guy. Steve was a retired man and did not charge for his services. He sometimes helped people who were experiencing extreme depression. He often worked with cancer patients. Kim's friend spoke very highly of him and said that he had helped her and several others. He called himself a Remote Viewer/Healer, but he was said to possess psychic abilities. Supposedly, he worked for the US Military when he was younger and would help them find spies. He saw things that others did not. His abilities are very much like those of psychic detectives.

A Psychic Detective[xxvii] is a person who investigates crimes by using purported paranormal psychic abilities. Examples have included post cognition (the paranormal perception of the past), psychometry (information psychically gained from objects), telepathy, dowsing, clairvoyance, and remote viewing. In murder cases, psychic detectives may purport to communicate with the spirits of the murder victims. I was surprised by two things. First, I was surprised that he could do his work over the phone. That seemed odd to me. Second, I was surprised that he did not charge for his services. This is what made me think that perhaps he might be for real. I took his phone number and promised Kim that I would watch the YouTube Videos and call Steve.

On June 29, we took the drive to Mayo and got my scans done early. While waiting for results, we picked up lunch for Ben which he ate in the car. I got oatmeal from Starbucks and picked at it. Later, Ben dropped me off at the entrance, and I got into a wheelchair and waited for him to park the car. I sat there and thought to myself that I should be able to walk by now. I should be able to do a lot of things for myself by now. Unfortunately, this was not how things were going for me. The worst part about my treatment was supposed to be the burns and fatigue. Something was wrong. Something was very wrong.

My first appointment was with Dr. Jordan. I had a bad case of 'scanxiety.' I weighed in at a whopping 106, and my blood pressure was 84/59. Jackie asked me how I was doing, and I told her that my chest pain was not any better. She was concerned by my demeanor. I was slumped over with my head resting on Ben's shoulder. I told her that I was still having trouble eating and gaining weight. It seemed to me that I was not digesting nutrients. She took notes. She asked me how my stools were, and I said they didn't hurt as much as they used to. She said that was good. She asked me if I was using the dilators, and I told her that I was not. I explained that it hurt too much. I was worried that I would close up down there, but I just could not use them. She wrote that down. She asked me which meds I was still on, and I told her that I was taking the max dosage of Prilosec every day and that it was not helping. I also told her that I took Lorazepam in the afternoon and at night.

When I told her that I had been to the ER three times, she looked concerned. She took more notes. I told her that I was worried about being put on a feeding tube. She wrote that down and asked me to take off my pants, sit on the examining table, and put a sheet on and that Dr. Jordan would be in soon to check my wounds. I was so worried about the results of my scan. She left the room, and I told Ben that I was terrified to get my results. Memories came rushing back to me about the last time Dr. Jordan gave me the results of a PET/CT scan. What made me think this was going to be good news? I had no reason to believe that. I felt like I had to prepare myself for the absolute worst. That would be that they did not get it all and that I had to have APR surgery. I was having a tough time breathing. I knew he was in another room close to this one, and he was looking over my scans with the radiologist. He would be coming into the room at any time now. I didn't think I could take any more bad news. I was already at a very low point.

I decided to hide in the dressing room. I sat up on the bench so that my feet would not show, and I pulled the curtain shut. Ben understood my fear. When Jackie came in with Dr. Jordan, they looked around and expected Ben to tell them that I was in the lady's room, but he pointed to the dressing room. After a minute or two, he told them that I was hiding in there because I was afraid of the scan results. Dr. Jordan asked me to come out and sit down. He said that he had good news for me. He told me that my scan showed that they got it all. He said that I responded very well to the treatments. I started to sob uncontrollably, and I hugged and thanked him. I hugged Ben too, and Jackie told me how happy she was for me. It was a huge relief. This could be the news that I needed. He did, however, have some bad news for me too. He said that he could no longer recommend me for the Opdivo trial. He said that I had too many side effects, and he didn't think it would be a good idea for me to be on an immunotherapy drug right now. I didn't even care at that point. I had to agree that I could not take another strong drug. I was way too weak. I knew that the deadline for getting into this trial would expire in a few days, so this was it. My opportunity to increase my odds for a complete cure was now history. I was on my own now and would not be getting into the clinical trial to prevent a recurrence. I would have to keep it from coming back on my own.

Dr. Jordan checked on my radiation areas and said that I was doing very well. He said that I should try my best to start the dilators soon but that I had time to let things heal for a bit. He told me to continue with the recommendations from Dr. Snyder and get the manometry test done. He said that if the Lorazepam was helping that I should continue as I have been. He told me that my blood tests looked good. I was overly concerned about my absolute lymphocytes because they were incredibly low. He said this was completely normal and that my white counts were stable overall. Dr. Jordan made it a point before he left the examination room to tell me that my odds just went from here to here. He used a flat hand to measure first down at mid-thigh and then up at just under his shoulders. He knew by now the effect that the original odds had on me and tried his best to right that wrong.

Ben told him that I was very depressed, and he asked me if I ever thought about suicide. This was something that they had to ask. I was honest and told him that I had but would never do it because of my kids. When he was finished with me, he told me to stay in the room and that a nurse would be coming in to ask me a few questions. A nurse came in after a few minutes, and she started to ask me questions about my depression and my suicidal thoughts. She said that she could not prescribe me anti-depressants but that I should see a psychologist to determine if I needed to be put on one. I told her that the news today would help me and that I could do this on my own. She was not satisfied. She told me that my insurance covered therapy and that she could get some recommendations for me. I said that I would consider that but that I would find someone in Prescott. She gave me her card and said she would follow up with me in a few days to make sure that I had.

We headed over to Medical Oncology and Dr. Li's office. Dr. Li's nurse came in and introduced herself as Susan. Susan started explaining procedures to me. She had zero bedside manner and zero empathy. She didn't ask me how I was doing but instead made it a point to tell me how long it would take her to respond to any calls or messages on the portal. If it were a weekday, I would get a response by the next business day, and if it was on the weekend, blah blah blah. Since I was a new patient of Dr. Li, she wanted me to understand their office procedures. I hated her. She must have known that I had complained about Dr. Kelson and Dr. Larkin not responding to me in a timely manner, and that was her way of setting me straight upfront with her and Dr. Li. Oh, that pissed me off. I later found this video online from an oncology nurse that got diagnosed with Colon Cancer. I wish I would have had it back then because I would have shown it to Susan. Here is what it said:

Dear every cancer patient I ever took care of, I'm sorry. I didn't get it.

This thought has been weighing heavy on my heart since my diagnosis. I've worked in oncology nearly my entire adult life. I started rooming and scheduling patients, then worked as a nursing assistant through school, and finally as a nurse in both the inpatient and outpatient settings. I prided myself in connecting with my patients and helping them manage their cancer and everything that comes with it. I really thought I got it - I really thought I knew what it felt like to go through this journey. I didn't.

I didn't get what it felt like to actually hear the words. I've been in on countless diagnoses conversations and even had to give the news myself on plenty of occasions but being the person the doctor is talking about is surreal. You were trying to listen to the details and pay attention, but really you just wanted to keep a straight face for as long as it took to maybe ask one appropriate question and get the heck out of there fast. You probably went home and broke down under the weight of what you had just been told. You probably sat in silence and disbelief for hours until you had to go pretend everything was fine at work or wherever because you didn't have any details yet and wanted to keep it private still. You probably didn't even know where to start, and your mind went straight to very dark places. That day was the worst. I'm sorry. I didn't get it.

I didn't get how hard the waiting is. It's literally the worst part. The diagnosis process takes forever. The different consults, the biopsies, the exams and procedures ... and the scans. Ugh, the scans. You were going through the motions trying to stay positive- but at that point, you had no idea what you were dealing with, and the unknown was terrifying. Knowing the cancer is there and knowing you're not doing anything to treat is yet an awful, helpless feeling. I'm sorry. I didn't get it.

I didn't get how awkward it was to tell other people the news. You didn't know what to say. They didn't know what to say. No one knew what to say- but there was some relief when the word started to spread. It may have been overwhelming to reply to all the calls and messages - and to get used to others knowing such personal information, but this nasty secret you'd been keeping was finally out, and your support system was growing. I'm sorry. I didn't get it.

I didn't get how much you hung onto every word I said to you. You replayed it in your mind a hundred times. Did I really mean this or that ... you wondered if you understood? You called me again to make sure. And maybe another time because your friend asked, "Well, what about ____?" You asked your other nurses to see if you got the same answer. Please know we are happy to take a million calls a day with the same questions until you can make sense of it. I'm sorry. I didn't get it.

I didn't get how much you googled. I told you not to do it. You did it, a lot- and so did I. Searching for information, hope, stories like yours, reassurance. It was impossible not to. My new stance is to just know what a good source is when you google. I'll help you learn to filter the information. And I promise to give you more information because I know how much you crave it. It's not realistic to think you will have the willpower to not search at all (at least it wasn't for me). I'm sorry. I didn't get it.

I didn't get what it felt like to get sad looks all the time. Walking down the hall at work or seeing someone for the first time after finding out. You got the head tilt with a soft "how aaaare you?" You quickly got together your rehearsed "Doing pretty good, tired but hanging in there" generic response. Don't get me wrong, I know you appreciated all the well wishes and concern - but it sure took a little while to get used to the pity. I'm sorry. I didn't get it.

I didn't get what really goes on at all those "other appointments." I knew what to tell you to expect at your oncology appointments- but all the different types of scans, radiation, operating room, procedural areas - I didn't really know what went on behind the scenes there and what to tell you. I should've known more about the whole picture. I should've been able to warn you that there was an hour wait after a dose of medication before you could actually have a scan. I should've been able to tell you what you can and can't eat or drink before a certain procedure or that some treatments require going every single day. I'm sorry. I didn't get it.

I didn't get how weird it felt to be called "brave." It's a word that gets thrown around a lot; yeah, it kind of made you feel good- but you still didn't really understand why people would call you this. Sure, you were getting through it fine (most days), but it's not like you had a choice. I'm getting treatment because I have to - it doesn't really make me feel like much of a hero. I'm sorry. I didn't get it.

I didn't get how crazy this makes you. Like you literally wondered if you had lost every working brain cell. Especially when dealing with side effects or other symptoms. You could've had every side effect in the book from chemo or none at all, and you'd still wonder if it's really working the way it's supposed to. You may just have had a headache, or a common cold, or a sore joint - but you were never certain it wasn't related to your cancer and always wondered if it was a sign of progression, even when it made no sense. I hope you didn't feel dismissed when you called me to ask about it, and I said not to worry. I'm sorry. I didn't get it.

I didn't get why you were always suspicious. You couldn't help but wonder if they all knew something you didn't about your prognosis. We shared the percentages and stats with you – and that every cancer is different ... but still- is there something more? Something they were protecting you from or just felt too bad to tell you? Logically, I know the answer to this but find myself with these feelings as well. I'm sorry. I didn't get it.

I didn't get how confusing "options" really were. In some cases, there may be more than one choice. Whether this be from physicians, medications, sequence of treatments, etc. - I would try my best to help you understand every angle, but more options many times just meant more confusion. You wanted to be involved in your own care - but the stress of too many options was sometimes too much. You begged me for my input and to tell you what I would do if it were me. I hated that question, but I hear you now. I'm sorry. I didn't get it.

I didn't get how hard it is to accept help. Especially the moms. This just wasn't something you're used to doing- but you needed it. You felt shy about admitting that you're not sure you could've gotten through the first few months without the extra food, gift cards, support, and other help you were given. You felt humbled at the outpouring and just only hoped you would've done the same for them. You still wonder if you said thank you enough or if you missed an opportunity to give back. I'm sorry. I didn't get it.

I didn't get the mood swings. One day you felt confident that you'd completely beat this with no problem; you felt like you could take over the world. And for no good reason, the next day you were just convinced yours was going to be one of those sad stories people tell their friends about. The moods snuck up on you without warning. Literally anything could've been a trigger. I'm sorry. I didn't get it.

I didn't get that when you said you were tired, you really meant so much more. Sure, there are words like exhaustion and extreme fatigue - but there should really be a separate word just for cancer patients, because it's crippling. Really. Some days you really wondered how you'd trudge forward. I'm sorry. I didn't get it.

I didn't get how much time this really takes away from your life. I always used phrases like "Cancer is like getting another full-time job" or "Life doesn't stop for cancer" when trying to prep you for what you were about to embark on. But now they just seem like corny catch phrases. It completely took over, you had to stop doing things you love, you had to cancel plans, you had to miss out on things that were important to you. It just wasn't in any plans - and that alone took a lot of mourning. I'm sorry. I didn't get it.

I didn't get how strange it was to see your body changing so quickly. You stood there and looked at yourself in disbelief in the mirror. Maybe it was extreme swelling; maybe it was the scars; maybe it was hair loss, maybe it was pounds melting away when you do everything in your power to eat as much as you can. It's hard - your appearance is tied more closely to your identity than you'd like to admit, and these were constant reminders of what you were up against. You just wanted to feel like yourself. I'm sorry. I didn't get it.

I didn't get that it hurts to be left out. People didn't invite you to things anymore. People felt like they can't complain or vent about everyday annoyances to you anymore. People acted differently towards you, and it hurt a bit. You certainly didn't blame them - you had even done the same to others when traumatic life events happened—and no, you didn't want to go out for drinks anyway because you don't feel good. But you needed normalcy. I'm sorry. I didn't get it.

I didn't get how much you worried about your kids. For this, I'm the most regretful. I should've talked to you more about them - and not just in terms of lifting restrictions or germs. You worried about how this was going to affect them. You worried about not being able to keep up with them or care for them properly on your bad days. You worried they'd be scared and confused. You worried about leaving them. I'm sorry. I didn't get it.

I didn't get the guilt you felt, especially to those who are married. You thought about how unfair it was that your spouse had to pick up so much slack - mentally to help keep you focused and calm and physically at home pulling double weight with never-ending everyday chores. You understood that everyone promises "in sickness and in health" when you get married- but you still felt like they didn't deserve this. You felt thankful when your spouse would say, "go get some rest, and I'll take care of the kids," but your heart hurt overhearing them play in the other room away from you - wondering if that was a glimpse into their future that didn't have you in it. I'm sorry. I didn't get it.

I didn't get that it never ends. Never. I used to tell you that cancer will be just a phase in your life. Just like high school or something - it seems like it drags on and on when you're in it, but soon it'll all be a memory. I'm sorry if this made you feel marginalized – it is not a phase. Yes, there are phases - the treatment won't last forever, but you are changed now. The worrying won't stop, the uncertainty won't stop, the fear of recurrence or an awful end won't stop. I hear that gets better - time will tell. And time is precious. I'm sorry. I didn't get it.

I do have to admit; I've probably had it a little easier than you to start off. I know the language, I know all the right people, I work where I get treatment, so, sure - it's more convenient. I watched so many of you march through this terrible nightmare with a brave face and determination- without knowing one thing about cancer ahead of time, other than knowing you didn't ever want to get it. You've always been my inspiration, and I love each and every one of you. Nothing brings me more joy than when I see you reach your goals and slowly put yourself back together. I love when we get visits or notes from those of you who are several years out and doing great - it's good for the oncology nurses' soul. Even though healthcare workers don't really know what it's like to be you (well, us), it's ok. Nobody does. I just hope that I was still able to give you a little guidance and strength to help you get through your cancer treatment, even if I didn't get it.

Love,
Lindsay, Oncology RN [xxviii]

When Dr. Li came in, he asked me how I was doing, but I did not feel like he listened to my answer. He made very little eye contact when speaking to me. Instead, his head was turned to his computer monitor. I could tell that he was confident and smart, but he did not have the patience to answer my questions. I expressed concern about my blood tests, and I wanted to know how long it would be before I could get back to doing things on my own. I also asked why I had these heartburn issues and how I was concerned my heart could be damaged. He told me that I had two of the strongest chemotherapy drugs on the market, equivalent to about 200 hours and that it could take a year before my fatigue subsided and that it could take years before my blood counts came back to normal. He told me matter-of-factly that, given the circumstances, they looked as they should. He then went on to tell me that I should be happy that I came through this as well as I did and that 1/3 of the patients don't make it through treatment. *I was stunned.* I had no idea. I guess he wanted me to be grateful and stop complaining. I didn't think I was complaining, but I asked many questions about why it took so long for me to feel better as compared to others. I thought to myself that he had no idea what I was going through and what right did he have to assume that all of this was from anxiety because probably that's what he was thinking. I was having genuine issues with chest pain, digestion, and fatigue, and he had absolutely no empathy for me. I told him that I worried that I could not gain weight and that the cancer would come back and that I would die a painful death from it. He had the nerve to tell me that I could die crossing the street and that I couldn't live my life in fear. Was he right about everything he said? Absolutely.

That night, I prayed to God and asked for my dad and my auntie. I told them that I missed them and needed them to help me get through this, but that if it was God's will that I should die, to please not let me die in pain. I was ready to go in my sleep and be with them again.

"I'm not afraid of dying. I just don't want to be there when it happens."

Woody Allen

Chapter 21

Awakening

I did not die in my sleep that night. The next morning, I called my kids and told them the good news about my scans. Ben's daughter usually came in for the Fourth of July every year, and I knew the grandkids wanted to come. She was waiting for me to give her the okay. I was not in any shape for company, but I knew that Ben needed to see them. I was leaning on him way too much, and he needed a break. His grandkids would be just the ticket. They would bring some much-needed joy to this home. I texted her and told her that it was okay for them to visit. She asked how I was doing, and I lied and told her that I was doing a little better.

Their visit was a bit hectic, but the kids gave me a reason to smile on several occasions. More than anything, I needed some joy in my life. When they first arrived, and they saw me, they came over to hug me. You could see that they were reluctant and curious. I am sure that their mom had prepared them in advance for my bald head and probably ensured that they would not be afraid to come up to me and hug me as was customary. I wondered what they thought. I showed them part of my shaved head from under my scarf, and they did not seem frightened by it.

They are highly active children. Allison is 11, Matt 10, and Mikey 5. One day they found out that they could set up a plastic ball on the rug in the family room with the patio doors open and take a full swing with the plastic child-size golf clubs in an attempt to get the ball to go over our back fence in the yard. The first ball went over the fence for the 5-year-old, and we all cheered for him. Then, of course, the others had to try. They are all into sports and incredibly competitive. Being the little athletes they are, they took turns trying to hit the whiffle ball over the fence. There were plenty of good shots that just missed and, of course, a fair share of swings and misses. Matt finally got one over, and we cheered. Then Mikey hit another one over. Poor Allison. She was the most talented athlete in the lot, and she could not get this stupid little plastic ball to go over the fence. We all knew that it was just dumb luck for the most part, but she was determined. I sat in my chair and laughed through it all until I saw Allison tear up a little after trying so hard and having to face the fact that her little brothers beat her at something. I tried to console her, but only time would heal that small wound.

They wanted me to come with them to the club pool and hit real golf balls at the driving range. They wanted me to go for rides in the golf cart at night to look for animals. They wanted me to go out to eat with them. They asked if I would join them in our hot tub at night and make s'mores at our fire pit afterward. They often stayed up late at night to watch a movie and eat popcorn. Mostly I heard the activity from my bed, but sometimes I came out to the recliner in the family room. Ben begged me to come with them to the pool one day, and so I did.

I put on my wig and a big sun hat and tried to hide how emaciated I looked by wearing a big cover-up over my suit. It was difficult to find a suit that even fit me. Carli offered to lend me one of hers, but I just put on a black one-piece that hung on me. I knew that I was never going to take off the cover-up anyway. I made it to the pool and sat in the shade. I saw a few people that I knew, and they came over and said how happy they were to see me out and about. I watched the kids and Ben playing in the pool and wondered when or if I would ever be back to normal. The sun's warmth felt good, but after about 45 minutes, I got very tired, so I took the golf cart home. Ben offered to take me home, but he was enjoying himself, so I left alone. It was enough for me. On another day, he talked me into driving out to the driving range with him and the kids. I put on some old bike shorts, a golf shirt, and a baseball hat and took the ride over. I sat on a bench and watched as the kids hit ball after ball, and I cheered them on for all their good shots. Ben had a challenging time keeping an eye on all three of them, so I think I helped. It felt good to be of some assistance instead of just a "slug." Ben talked me into hitting a couple of balls. That was so much effort on my part, but I hit three perfect shots. It was weird, but I had a slow swing, and my head stayed down. This is perfect for golf. One of the biggest mistakes that golfers often make is trying to muscle the ball. You must swing slow and let the club do the work, and you have to keep your head still and finish your swing. I was a little tired, and Ben had enough, so we cut the trip short. He could take them again later, as they had endless energy. I asked the kids on the way home if they could lend me just an ounce of their energy. They said, "Sure, grandma."

Maybe I pushed myself a little too hard because later, I had a bad night of shaking and chest pains. I felt very bloated and tried to sit up in bed for as long as I could. Ben felt bad for me. The kids wanted their Paca to play with them, and he knew that I needed him that night. After they went to bed, I got worse. I took my pills, and nothing was helping. Finally, I started to get very emotional, and Ben said we should go to the ER. I put it off as long as possible, but we ended up going at about five am.

We were both exhausted, and the place was packed. It was a holiday weekend. Holidays are always busy in the ER. I got in for my usual EKG, and it was normal. I waited again while broken bones and overdoses were tended to. There was an older man who looked like he was ten shades of red. They took him in quickly. By the time they took me in, I had thrown up and felt a little better. I went in anyway, and they gave me some IV hydration and some pain meds. It amazed me that of the six times I visited this ER, I have had a different doctor every time and a distinct set of nurses. This time we were gone for a full seven hours. I slept for a good part of the next day, and Ben tried to function as best he could with the kids. Carli felt like they were imposing, and she did everything possible to make herself helpful. I did not want her or the kids to ever feel like they are imposing on us. They made me focus on something other than my illness for a few days, and that was huge.

After they left, our house became eerily quiet. It was always like that when the grandkids left. It's like a hurricane when they are here, and then when they leave, you can hear crickets. I now had plenty of time to dwell on my feelings again. I started to have some "good days," but that is probably an overstatement. By far, most of my days were still quite challenging. Ben was gone a lot, and I slipped back into my dark place. I just did not want to live like this anymore. I tried to cook a meal, and I would get as far as taking a few things out of a cabinet. I tried to clean up after myself, and the most I could do would be to bring a dish into the sink. I didn't even have the strength to stand up for the time it took to wash the dish. I left the slider open so that the dogs could come in and out as they pleased. They bark at everything, and sometimes it got excessive, especially when our neighbors let their dog Lucy out at the same time. Our dogs began barking, and I did not have the strength to get them back in. I had to listen to them bark on some days for what seemed like hours. I was just waiting for someone to call the police on them. This stressed me out even more than I already was. I was getting tired of living like this. This was not living to me.

I decided to look into the Joe Dispenza You Tube videos. In one of his videos, he talks about how our thoughts have consequences so great that they can create our reality. What we think and believe has a profound effect on our world. Our past experiences are dangerous when they include strong feelings of anger, guilt, shame, and vengeance. When we feel these negative emotions, adrenaline can pump, the heart can race, and blood pressure can rise. This is a natural response more commonly known as the 'fight or flight' mode. This is important when we are faced with immediate danger, however, we can get stuck in this mode for unnecessary, prolonged periods and that can result in suppression of the immune system. He believes that the power of the mind is so great that negative energy can affect our physical bodies. Conversely, he believes that we have the power to heal ourselves by changing that thought process.

I decided to call Steve. I left a detailed message for him and told him I was friends with the owner of the Crystal Shop. He called me back within the hour. I was at a very low point when I spoke to him. He got right to the matters at hand. He asked me what was going on, and I told him about my cancer and the doctor's odds. He said, "He did what? "

He was angry that my doctor said that to me. He asked me a lot more questions and wanted to know how I was feeling. I told him that I wanted to die. I told him that I could not live like this much longer and that the only thing stopping me was my kids. He asked about my family, my husband, my life, and any unresolved issues that I might be holding onto. He wanted to know if there were any other times in my life that I experienced depression. I told him about my depression after my divorce and how I never really worked through it. I told him that Ben was a good man but that he was not the type to listen to my feelings. I told him how difficult it was for me to enjoy my life after that. I never really expressed those feelings to anyone before. Then I told him about my diagnosis and how I was convinced that it was a punishment and that it was slowly killing me. I felt that I had done nothing special with my life and that everyone would eventually just forget about me. He asked me to get a journal and write letters to anyone that I had any unresolved issues with and get them resolved!

"Just write it all out like you are having a conversation with them, then burn it. Put it in your fireplace, fire pit, or wherever, and burn it. Watch the smoke and flames until they are gone. If you want to call them, then call them on the phone, but you don't have to. You can just write it all down."

Then he told me some very odd things. He told me that I had several past lives and that I came from another planet originally. He called the planet, Zircon. He said Zircon had to be evacuated because it got too hot for life and the population scattered to various places.

I went to Earth, and my fairy came with me. He said that my fairy meant well but gave me bad advice based on the energy from the other planet. The other planet did not operate on the same wavelengths as Earth, and she was harming me by staying with me. He excused himself from our conversation and started to speak directly to her. He asked her to please let me go because she was killing me. I cried. I don't know why. It was so absurd, but it was also so real. I wanted desperately to believe. He said that she agreed and wished me only the best. He then went on to heal me. He went through every part of my body. He did not talk to me anymore. He spoke directly to the creator. He first asked for time from the creator, and then he told me that the creator granted him time. He asked the creator if he would clear my blood from all toxins, and it was granted. He asked the creator if he would clear my heart and other organs from all toxins, and it was granted. He went on and on for every part of my body until he finally got to my immune system. He made a point to concentrate on this area because he knew that I was concerned about my cancer coming back. He asked the creator to bring my immune system back to its optimal strength, and his request for me was granted. The last step was to ask for my mental health to return to how it was before my divorce and my sickness. It was granted.

Before we ended the call, he told me he did what he could but that the rest was up to me. He said that I HAD to believe that I was healed. I had to believe it with every cell in my body. I cried, and I believed. As crazy as it all was, I believed. It's all you can do when nothing else is working. You find something to believe in. He told me that I did not have to believe in God, but I needed to believe in something greater than myself. He sometimes called the creator God. I think it meant the same thing to him. Immediately after I ended the call with Steve, a huge weight lifted from me. I can't explain it. It just happened.

I then began my letters. This took me a few days. I started by writing to my mother. When I was six years old, my mother died, and I may have felt some anger toward her for how she treated my oldest sister. I told her that after she punished them, my sisters would then take it out on me. I told her that I forgave her and understood that she did not mean to hurt us. I also forgave her for leaving us so early without a mother. I told her that I was sorry that she got sick and that she had such a short life, and I told her that I loved her.

I wrote to my dad and told him that I understood why he got so mean to me in his later years. I said that I knew that it was his dementia speaking to me and not really him. I said that I missed him a lot and that I would remember him like he used to be and not how he was in the end. I said that I knew how much pain he was in and was glad that he was no longer hurting. I told him about the pain I was in now and that I was not ready to join him yet. I explained to him that I needed to be around to help Tony and Michelle but that I would see him and mommy someday soon. I said how happy I was that they were together again. I thanked him for being both a mother and father to me and always being such a good role model. I told him how much I loved him and could not have asked for a better father. I also said that I would make up with my sisters. I knew that he wanted that from me more than anything else.

I wrote to my oldest sister, Barb. I told her that I understood why she never had a good relationship with her daughter. I wrote that it must be hard for her to deal with the things that happened in her past. I knew that I only saw the tip of the iceberg as far as the fights with my mom went. She got the brunt of mom's anger. I forgave her for treating my niece Robin the same way. I told her that I always felt that she had it the hardest growing up and that I loved her. I promised to check in on her a lot more often.

I wrote to my sister Marnie, and this was a hard letter to compose. I still held resentment toward her for turning my dad against me right before he died. I told her that I believed that if she did take the money, she deserved it. For many years, I did not have to worry about my dad as much because she came to visit him on the weekends. I told her that I did not care about the money. Money could not buy my health right now, so what good was it. I told her how much fun I had with her when we were rehabbing my dad's condominium and that I missed being close with her. I told her that I was sorry for not calling her more often, and I regret how we have grown apart over the years. We should have done more together as a family when our kids were young. I wrote that she could come to me whenever she needed to vent about taking care of her husband and that I loved her and would be there for her.

I then wrote a letter to my ex-husband. This was another toughie. I told him how sorry I was for lying to him. I should have communicated better, and I should have insisted on therapy long before our infidelities. I told him that he was my best friend for most of my life and that I would never forget those years. I said that we made some great kids together and that we will always have that. I forgave him for everything I could think of and apologized for just as much.

I wrote a heart-wrenching letter to my son. To Tony, I said he needed to know that I loved him more than my own life. I wanted more than anything for him to get his life together and for him to stop drinking and find a partner and have a healthy, stable, and happy life. I apologized for not being the parent that I should have been. I apologized for breaking up our family and told him that I knew how hard he took that. I told him that I always loved him and felt proud of him even when he acted impulsively and made mistakes. He is emotional, generous, and he is my one-in-a-million son.

To Michelle, I wrote that she stole my heart when she was born and that I was proud of her accomplishments. I told her how much I appreciated her coming to my rescue when I needed her before and during treatment. I apologized to her also for my breaking up our family, and I hoped she would forgive me. I told her that I loved her more than words could express. I hoped she would be happy in her relationship and reconsider having children of her own someday, but that I would support her decision either way. I said that I thought she would make a great mom.

Lastly, I wrote a long letter to Ben. I wanted him to know how much he has helped me throughout my illness. I told him that at first, I was angry that I might have gotten the HPV virus from him. I explained my feeling that this was the ultimate punishment for my affair with him. I admitted that I wondered how I would be able to live with him knowing that I may have contracted the HPV from him. I told him about the woman from Chicago who had never been with any other man but her husband and how angry she was with him. My letter went on to say that I knew from my research that this HPV could lay dormant in my body for years, so it could have come from anyone in my past. I said that even if it was from him, I was not angry about it any longer. I know that it was not intentional in any way. I said that I was sorry for mistrusting him in the past and that I was lucky to have him in my life. I told him that my plan had always been to take care of him when he got older. I apologized for that plan not working out. I said that I knew that he was doing a lot for me right now and that I would make up for it someday. My letter said that I could not have survived any of this without him by my side and that even though he did not express it often, I could finally feel how much he loved me.

I also wrote short notes to several other friends, relatives, and doctors. In the end, I promised to treat those same people with love and respect regardless of past disagreements. It would benefit no one to hold onto old grudges. I had to let it all go.

I took all the papers and had a little ceremony in my backyard fire pit. I watched as the flames turned to dark smoke and then sparked and filtered into the air until they were just ash floating in the wind.

I spent the next few weeks working on my mental health. Steve gave me a lot to think about and taught me the power of positivity and faith.

I was already going to acupuncture two to three times per week, but I needed more help. I promised the nurse at Mayo that I would see a therapist, and shortly she would be checking up on me to see that I had done just that. I decided to interview a few just to make sure I had a connection with the person. I asked the first therapist a few questions about the types of patients she worked with. I got the impression that she was best at family counseling.

The second therapist I saw was working out of her home on the outskirts of town. Her house was on a big lot and included a horse barn. I knew in advance that she used horses as part of her therapy. We talked for a bit in her house and then walked out to a corral where a large horse was grazing. She introduced me to Whisper and asked me to lie on a reclining lawn chair. She called Whisper over and pulled him down toward me. She told me where to touch him and warned me about a couple of things he did not like. I was nervous around Whisper and knew instantly that this therapy was not for me. That was one huge horse.

The third was a small-framed German lady with a heavy accent. Her name was Simone. Simone shared an office with a massage therapist. Her side of the office was very private and opened onto a beautiful courtyard. There were comfortable chairs, a couch, and her desk. It was far from clinical looking, and she had several photos of children on her desk, which I assumed were her grandchildren. She was dressed casually and wore wide lilac linen slacks and Birkenstock sandals. I asked if she specialized in any areas of mental health. She was honest and told me that most of her current clients came from the various rehab facilities that Prescott is famous for. She said that she has been practicing for over thirty years, so she has seen her share of various clients. She had worked with addicts, vets with PTSD, couples, families, and even disaster victims. After I told her about my diagnosis and treatment, she told me she could help me with my depression and anxiety. She hit the nail right on the head. I told her that I wanted to set up a session, and she took my insurance information and planned on one hour per week to start.

My manometry appointment was scheduled for the next day, and after much deliberation, I decided to cancel it. I was just starting to have a few decent days here and there, and I did not want to have a tube down my throat day and night. I was still only 107 pounds and struggling to eat. I was at a point where I would get hopeful after a good day, and then the next day would be terrible, and I would get shot down. My body would slap me back to reality, and I would have another setback. It was often one step forward and two steps back! I changed my mind at the last minute and decided to reschedule it two weeks later instead of canceling.

Lastly, I decided to buy another ten passes for the Photon Genius Infrared Sauna and the Photo Genie Radio Frequency. I planned to alternate between the two. My days were full between the Photon Genius, Photo Genie, acupuncture, naturopath, integrative physician, primary care physicians, and oncologists. I didn't have time to sit around and feel sorry for myself. I even started to go on some short shopping trips with Ben. I could make a short trip to CVS or The Natural Grocer because they were small stores. The Natural Grocer was an independent store where I could get organic produce and dry goods. They also had a large section of supplements, which was handy when I forgot to order something online. I started back on my juicing and supplement program, so we made frequent trips to the store for fresh produce. I wanted to go to Frye's to help Ben pick out groceries that I would eat, but I hesitated because of the area I would need to cover. He reminded me that they have the electric scooters with the shopping carts attached.

"Hell Ya," I said, "I can do that."

I just hoped that I would not see anyone I knew. My first experience was quite interesting. I was by far the youngest and thinnest occupant of the motorized shopping cart vehicles. Ben took a video of me on my first mission. It took a little getting used to. After that, I became a pro and could be seen frequenting Walmart and Costco too. I fit right in at Walmart!

My first appointment with Simone was primarily a get to know one another session. She asked me a lot of questions about my family and Ben. She wanted to know about my parents and where I grew up. We talked about family and friends. When I started to get into more serious topics, she pulled me back to get more background information. On my second appointment, she could tell that I was not feeling well, so we talked about my current health issues. There was no way to discuss my current health issues without getting into my whole story. I started to cry when I discussed my diagnosis. She handed me the tissues. I explained to her that I was having GI pain and that it felt like I was having a heart attack when it got bad. I could only explain it as a tightness or heaviness in my chest. I told her that I had been to the emergency room six times during and after my treatment ended. She was a good listener. Our one-hour appointments went by so quickly. When it was time for me to leave, Simone always wanted a big hug.

I got a call from a nurse at Mayo. She was checking on me to see if I had set up the therapy. She caught me on a difficult day. I told her that I had just started and that I was happy with my choice. She asked me several other questions, including the one about wanting to end my life. I was honest, and I told her the truth. I told her that most of my days were bad and that when I had a good one, I would get hopeful that my health was turning a corner. Then, the next morning, I would wake up in pain, and the hope would turn to dread. I told her that I was doing everything I could to make myself get out of the house and do things but was still struggling. I further explained that I was having a hard time gaining any weight and experiencing frequent gastrointestinal issues. She asked if I was following up with Dr. Snyder, and I said that I was. I explained that I had a Manometry test coming up. She asked again about my mood, and I told her that at night, I sometimes prayed (and I wasn't a particularly religious person) that God would take me in my sleep. I started to cry, and she said that I should see Dr. Bright at Mayo when I came down for my Manometry test. She would set up an appointment for me, hopefully for that same day. I agreed to see him.

On the day of my Manometry test, Ben had a tournament, and I was having an okay day. He said that he would cancel his tournament and take me to Mayo, but I knew how much golf meant to him, and I told him that I was feeling fine and insisted on going myself. On the ride down, I played music and contemplated my life. I also thought about the patients that did not make it through the initial treatment. I felt sorry for them but also wondered if they might be the lucky ones. If this was my new life, I wanted no part of it. At Mayo, I first met with a nurse in the room where the Manometry equipment would be set up. The first thing she did was to show me the tubing. I looked at one and said, "that's not bad," and she explained that the small one pulled this other one through. She then showed me the tube that would be pulled through my nose and down into my stomach for a whole weekend. She showed me the monitor that I would wear clipped on my pants. Oh shit! That tube looked so thick! I could not imagine having that in one of my nostrils 24/7. She then pulled up a lengthy questionnaire and explained the test to me. She said that the Esophageal Manometry test would measure the function of my lower esophageal sphincter. That is the valve that prevents reflux. In layman terms, the test measures the ability of my esophagus to move food to my stomach properly. I would not be sedated for the insertion of the tube. I would receive just a topical anesthetic to my nose. Oh Jeez! I was getting more and more nervous about this test. She said it was possible that I would cough or vomit during the procedure. She started to ask me questions. No. 1. Was I having difficulty swallowing? No. 2. Did I have pain when swallowing? No. 3. Did I regurgitate my food or bring it back up after swallowing? No. 4. Did I experience heartburn or acid reflux? I don't know. 5. Did I experience non-cardiac chest pain? I guess so. 6. Did I cough a lot, especially after eating? No. 7. Did I experience nausea after eating? Sometimes. The questionnaire also contained a consent form and warnings about the procedure. Call your doctor immediately or go to the nearest emergency room if any of the following occur:

✓ A fever of 101 or higher
✓ Difficulty Swallowing
✓ Pain in Your Chest
✓ Stomach Pain, Hardness or Bloating
✓ Nausea or Vomiting
✓ Severe or constant Bleeding from your Nose
✓ Any Unexpected or Unexplained other Problems

The nurse told me that the biggest complication would be if I got an infection from the tubing. There was always a chance of that. Then she asked if I was nervous about the test. I said that I was and that I was concerned because I answered No to most of the questions and that I had a strong feeling that this test would just add to the problems that I already had, like not being able to eat. She said I should not feel like I had to proceed with the procedure if I did not feel right about it. She said that most patients had difficulty swallowing, and I told her that it was never difficult for me. She said it would be no problem at all if I decided to cancel the test. She would just tell the doctor that I decided against it. I thanked her and left.

I went all that way to Mayo and backed out of the test. I had to be on an empty stomach for the test, so I drank a bottle of water and headed over to the Shea Street hospital for my Psychiatry appointment. Dr. Bright was a good-looking middle-aged man who wore a bow tie. Only certain people could wear bow ties. He was one of them. I imagined that he wore them all the time and had several at home to choose from. He could tell from my demeanor that I was depressed. I thought he would ask a few questions and prescribe me an anti-depressant, which would be the end of it. That's what I was there for. He was nothing like I expected. He started by asking me how I was doing, and I explained that I was post-treatment for Anal Cancer, and he wanted to hear all about what I had been through.

I explained the treatment and how I thought that based on others who had been through the same, by now, I would be getting better. I told him that I had a plan to go on a serious naturopathic protocol right after treatment ended and that because of unplanned side effects, I could not implement that plan. I felt that I was way behind schedule and that the cancer would return. I started to cry, and he handed me the tissue box. I also didn't understand why I cried so much. He asked me more about that. I explained that I cried almost all the time when I was alone. He asked me about my childhood, and I told him that I had a happy childhood and did not understand why I was so depressed. He asked if I had ever experienced depression before in my life, and I told him that I had, after my divorce, but it was not as constant as this. He pressed again to learn more about my childhood. I told him that my mother died when I was six and that I had been molested a couple of times and experienced a date rape when I was young and one time at knifepoint.

Dr. Bright stopped me and said, "You are going through this list like it is nothing," and I said, "Well, compared to some of my friends, it IS nothing."

He told me to stop comparing myself to others. He told me that what happened to me WAS important and that it impacted my life. He said that all my experiences had an impact on my life. I explained that I got the most emotional when I thought about getting my cancer back again. I explained how I felt that I should be happy the treatment worked and that my scans were clear. Yet, all I kept thinking was that it would come back again, and I would die a painful death from this. I cried some more. I explained that I thought it might be coming from the diagnosis I got from Dr. Jordan when he first gave me my staging and odds for recovery. I explained to Dr. Bright that I was sorry that I had even asked for those odds. I told him that I needed to know them to decide on my method of treatment. I was really against chemo and radiation. I strongly believed that I could do this without conventional treatment. I believed that I could heal myself through nutrition and by improving my immune system. I told him that Dr. Jordan gave me a 30 percent chance of curing my cancer and upped that to 50 percent if I had APR surgery.

I cried some more. I must have looked like a total wreck. I had put on makeup that morning, and I now had mascara running down my face. I explained how Dr. Jordan staged me as 3C, and I was not expecting it. I was not expecting any of it because I felt great prior to treatment. I had never been in a hospital in my life before this except to have my children. I talked about my children. He asked me more about my mother and what had happened to me as a child, and my divorce. We then came back again to my current situation. He said that I had a form of PTSD. I said that I thought that was something that veterans got from combat, and he explained that it affected many people who had been through tragedies, and I had certainly been through the tragedy of losing my health and that I had just gone through a very painful treatment regime. I explained how Dr. Jordan told me that he had to "hit it hard." Those were words that I could not forget. I told him how one-third of patients do not make it through the initial treamtment and that I should be grateful for being alive.

Dr. Bright had my file, and he knew the extent of my treatment. He said that I had gotten over 200 hours of chemo in just eight days. I never thought of it that way before. Many cancer patients get their chemo in much lower doses over many months or years. I also had two of the oldest and strongest chemo drugs ever made. He told me that I had to stop discounting what I went through and stop discounting what I was currently going through. It would take time for my body to heal from all of that. He felt that I should not have to go through this recovery period without feeling some happiness. He wanted to put me on a low dose of Lexapro. He said that the drug has been around a long time and that it was proven safe and effective and that I would not become dependent on it. He suggested a 3-month prescription just to get me through this rough patch. He knew how I felt about medications, and he explained it well. Unfortunately, it would take a few weeks to start working, so he suggested that I start today if possible. I told him that I would.

I told him that I saw a therapist in Prescott and liked her but that we were just getting started. He asked me if she had any experience with EMDR therapy.[xxix] I did not know what that was. He said it was a therapy used with PTSD patients that worked with the two sides of the brain and helped patients process their trauma. He wanted me to understand that my physical and emotional pain was real, and my fears of a relapse intensified it and that I needed to get that from one side of my brain to the other. I didn't really understand all of it. He gave me a list of therapists in the area who practiced EMDR therapy. Unfortunately, they were all in the Phoenix area. I said that I would investigate it, and I said that I would also fill the prescription. Dr. Bright lived up to his name, and I was glad that I went to see him.

I made the long drive back to Prescott and stopped at CVS on the way home to pick up the Lexapro. I started on it immediately. When I told Ben about canceling the manometry procedure, he said that he was glad. I could always reschedule it again if things did not improve.

I saw a friend from the club the next morning when I was getting my mail, and she asked how I was doing. I said that I was "hanging in there." She said that she heard that I was not doing well and having a tough time eating. I said that was true and that I was doing my best to get through it. I asked her what else she had heard at the club? What were others saying about me? She said that one woman said my problems were from anxiety. I was livid! I told her that I had a strong treatment and that I had real pain and that anxiety was also a very real medical issue, and that I was doing my best to get through both. I told her thanks for being concerned and took my mail and left. I was really hurt, thinking that others were dismissing my pain as anxiety. I felt that I was just another reason for some folks to gossip. I should not care what people say about me behind my back, but I did, and it hurt my feelings that others were judging me.

Well, my friends from high school were coming to town to celebrate our 60th birthdays. *Oh great! They were coming to see me, and I felt like shit.* Fran, the organizer, was coming in from Seattle and had rented a big house in Prescott. Leah and

Carol were coming in from Chicago, and Dar was coming in from Memphis. Sue was coming in from Phoenix and Mindy from Alaska. Mindy insisted on staying with me. All the rest were staying at the rental house. Mindy and her husband and three boys moved to Anchorage many years ago for work reasons. I visited them once after the tragic death of their oldest son. When he was just 19 years old, he took his life. Mindy has not been the same since. She turned to God for her salvation, and it has helped her immensely. She even took a trip to Lourdes, France, where approximately 7000 people have claimed to have experienced miracles. Of those 7000, over 70 have been classified as scientifically unexplainable.

It all began in 1858 when it is said that a 14-year-old girl saw the Virgin Mary in a cave. It is now a huge tourist destination. Mindy brought everyone a bracelet from Lourdes, and to me, she also brought a container of the holy water. I grew up in a religious family and went to a catholic grade school and a catholic all-girl high school. I was baptized, had my first communion and confirmation, and have had my children baptized. My first marriage was held in a catholic church, and we even went to pre-Cana classes before we were married. Somewhere in my late twenties, I stopped going to church and fell out of step with my religion, but deep down, I still believed in some aspects of it. I believed strongly in many of the morals that were taught to me. I believed in faith. For example, the scriptures have taught me to 'turn the other cheek,' and that 'the meek shall inherit the earth,' and to 'practice what you preach,' and that we should have 'respect for our elders,' and 'honesty is the best policy,' and 'do unto others as you would have them do unto you,' and of course the ten commandments.

I've broken a few of them, but I do believe that they are rooted in me. One of the things people often make fun of about

Catholics is that we are taught to feel guilt and shame over our indiscretions. I think that's true.

Anyway, I agreed to go to church with Mindy on Sunday. We have one catholic church in Prescott, and we went there for their 11 am Mass. We sat in the back, and I felt welcome and comfortable. I did love the feeling that being in church gave me–the smell of the incense, the beautiful altar, and statues. I asked for forgiveness for my sins and prayed for others who were suffering. Mindy took communion and insisted that I could also do so, but I had been taught that you don't take communion if you have not had formal confession, so I did not join in the Sacrament of the Eucharist. I looked around at the congregation and felt like part of a community being around them. I could fully understand why people were drawn to religion. For me, it was a big part of my childhood, and even though I no longer attended church, it will forever be ingrained in my life.

I am unsure what meds Mindy was on, but she was super high energy, and mine was completely depleted. She wanted to swim, hike, bike, and work out. She wanted to go shopping, and she could stay in the stores forever. She asked endless questions, and I tried but could not keep up. We insisted she stay in our casita so that the dogs would not bark as much, but they still barked every time she came in and out of the house. It was like having the grandkids all over again. There were many times when I just told her to take my car and go so that I could get some rest. I must admit that she didn't allow me to wallow, but she also didn't allow me to rest.

We all went to our pool at the club one afternoon, and I treated cocktails and appetizers. I sat back and watched as they swam and got loaded. The plan was to go downtown after, so I tried to walk through the town with them. I got tired very quickly and had Ben pick me up. The next day, they told me how much fun they had in one of the bars. I guess they had a great band and they danced and drank all night. I must admit that I was envious that I could not partake in the festivities. There was drama also; there is always drama. It was like high school all over again. Some of the girls were fighting about this and that. Fran got into it with Mindy about insisting that she stay with me. Fran told her that if she was going to stay with me, she needed to help me and not cause me more stress. Mindy was insulted and took it wrong. Then Carol got involved. Both Carol and Mindy had Breast Cancer, so in many ways, they knew what it was like to be me right now, or they thought they did. It was a huge mess. Our friend Sally had a dinner planned at her house in Prescott Valley. She and her husband had just retired here from California and had a brand-new house they wanted everyone to visit. We all went except Mindy. She was over an hour late from a shopping trip, so we all went without her. It was an enjoyable time, but again, I left early and then had to listen to Mindy complain the rest of the evening.

Finally, everyone except Carol left Prescott. Carol came to stay with me for a few more days. She overlapped with Mindy for one day, and they got into a big fight. They mentioned shit that was 30 years old. It made no sense to me at all. I tried to stay out of it. The last three days with Carol were fine. We talked a lot about depression because she had also been through her share of it. She was also seeing a therapist, and she felt that it helped her a great deal. Here I was trying to avoid pain pills and anti-depressants at a time when they were medically necessary, and most of my closest friends were self-medicating to avoid the pain in their lives. I was beginning to realize that we all had problems in our lives, and it reminded me of a quote: "If we all tossed our problems into a pile and saw everyone else's, we'd grab ours back." That could be true, even in my case.

On my next appointment with Simone, I told her about my appointment with Dr. Bright at Mayo and how he put me on Lexapro and asked her if she ever used EMDR therapy. She said that she had but that it had been a while. She said that she would be happy to try it with me. I asked her to explain it, and she said that it was a therapy used with often superior results in people that have experienced trauma. She explained that EMDR stood for Eye Movement Desensitization and Reprocessing. She told me that practitioners usually took one of three approaches. Most used lateral eye movement approaches, thus the name. Some used hand-tapping, and still others used the audio stimulation approach. Her experience was with the latter. She would put a set of headphones on me and play calming music that would shift from one ear to the next. She further explained that it was a psychotherapy treatment designed to alleviate the distress associated with traumatic memories. The Adaptive Information Processing model posits that EMDR therapy facilitates the accessing and processing of traumatic memories and other adverse life experiences to bring these to an adaptive resolution. After successful treatment with EMDR therapy, affective distress is relieved, negative beliefs are reformulated, and physiological arousal is reduced. During EMDR therapy, the client attends to emotionally disturbing material in brief sequential doses while simultaneously focusing on external stimuli.

In layman terms, EMDR is a psychotherapy that enables people to heal from the symptoms and emotional distress resulting from disturbing life experiences. Repeated studies show that by using EMDR therapy, people can experience the benefits of psychotherapy that once took years to make a difference. It is widely assumed that severe emotional pain requires a long time to heal. EMDR therapy shows that the mind can heal from psychological trauma, much like the body recovers from physical trauma. I am all about that quick fix and helping the body do what it is naturally inclined to do. When you cut your hand, your body works to close the wound. If a foreign object or repeated injury irritates the wound, it festers and causes pain. Once the block is removed, healing resumes.

More than thirty positive controlled outcome studies have been conducted on EMDR therapy. Some studies show that 84-90% of single-trauma victims no longer have post-traumatic stress disorder after only three 90-minute sessions. Another study, funded by the HMO Kaiser Permanente, found that 100% of the single-trauma victims and 77% of the multi-trauma victims no longer were diagnosed with PTSD after only six 50-minute sessions. In another study, 77% of combat veterans were free of PTSD in 12 sessions. There has been so much research on EMDR therapy that it is now recognized as an effective form of treatment for trauma and other disturbing experiences by organizations such as the American Psychiatric Association, the World Health Organization, and the Department of Defense. Given the worldwide recognition as an effective treatment of trauma, you can easily see how EMDR therapy would effectively treat the "everyday" memories that cause people to have low self-esteem, feelings of powerlessness, and a myriad of problems that bring them in for therapy. Millions of people have been treated successfully over the past 25 years. I can't believe that this is the first time I heard about this. I can think of a lot of people that could use it.

We decided together that this approach warranted merit for me and that we would try this at our next therapy session.

The next week went by quickly. I still had bad days and good ones. Ben was trying to get me to start golfing again, but I wasn't ready. What if I had to use the bathroom in an emergency. How embarrassing would that be? What if I couldn't play more than a few holes and got tired. He said I could just play with him. So, when the course was empty in the late afternoon, we took the dogs out in the golf cart (they stayed in the cart), and he watched me play a couple of holes. It wasn't much, but it was something. I was hitting the drives about 120 yards, which was a far cry from what I was used to. But I was out there and trying.

It was Thursday again, and I drove myself to Simone's office. She handed me a pair of headphones, and I put them on. We adjusted the sound so that I could still hear her talk to me when I had them on. The music was instrumental and strange to me. It was called binaural and was said to contain certain healing tones. It came in rhythmic patterns, switching from my left ear to my right ear with variating volume levels.

Simone already knew me pretty well, so she started by asking me how I felt when Ben went golfing and left me alone. This did not elicit a strong response. I told her that it used to be a problem for us in the past when I thought that he was putting his own desires ahead of my feelings after my divorce. She asked me more about my divorce, and I told her that I had felt a great deal of guilt for breaking up our family and that my son's issues with alcohol were my fault. I got very emotional about that, and she talked me through it, explaining that I was only human and that I needed to forgive myself. I told her that I understood that I should get past those feelings. I think she started me off with smaller traumas to see how I reacted to the bigger ones.

She then touched on the trauma I experienced when I was 11 and how I felt about that. I told her about the rape and other incidents in my past. I told her that I thought I might have a strong dislike for certain men, and she said that I probably had a fear of men's sexuality and that I should know that most men do not force themselves on women and that I could trust them. We talked about my feelings of insecurity due to losing my mother at such a young age. I told her how I did not have any close friends to talk with about my feelings and that Ben was not the type to have any deep conversations with. I told her how I often felt left out and that I thought people did not like me. I told her how seldom I smiled or laughed anymore and how I wished that I could go back in time to when I was much happier.

We discussed how sensitive I was to certain feelings of abandonment and how this was a natural response to losing my mother at such a young age. Then she found a weak spot. It had to do with why I got HPV. I got very emotional when I started to discuss my sexual encounters with men. It seems that I did not blame them like I thought. I blamed myself. I also felt like my cancer was a punishment. I verbalized this many times to my doctors. I wasn't sure why I felt this way or who was punishing me. I blamed myself for starting a relationship with Ben while I was still married. I blamed myself for the rape because I did not fight harder to stop it. I got all of this out, and I told her that I knew it was not my fault but that I still felt that I would do things much differently if I could go back.

She reminded me of the statistics of HPV in the population and how young I was when I was molested. Also, losing my mother at such an early age could have prevented me from learning many valuable lessons, which I instead had to learn independently. She said that I should forgive myself and love myself, and I cried like a baby. We went over the session time, and she hugged me on the way out. All the while we talked, I listened to the music playing in the background and going from one side of my head to the next and changing volumes. It was quite interesting. We planned to pick up where we left off next week.

I decided to try golfing on a Tuesday with my former group. It was a bad idea. My tee shots were, on average, 50 yards shorter than anyone else's. My driver used to be my favorite club. I also hit a lot of ground balls and shanks. I just had no focus anymore. I had to bring my butt pillow with me because the cart was so bumpy, and I often stopped at the restroom. I prayed that I would not have an accident while I was with them. I used the excuse to ride alone because I might get tired and leave early, but really, I was worried about having uncontrollable gas or, even worse, diarrhea. It was too embarrassing for me to even discuss with anyone. So far, this had happened only at home, but what if it happened when I was out? It was discouraging, but I made it through the round. The girls insisted that they would hold this spot for me, but I no longer felt like I fit in. I did not voice my feelings.

When I was in treatment, another girl took my spot and I felt like they preferred playing with her. I felt like all I talked about was my cancer or treatments, but that was my life for the last several months. They liked to make small wagers, and I could no longer compete. They even changed the game to make it easier for me. I wanted to quit. Ben told me that I needed to give myself a break and that people understood and sympathized with me. I stuck it out for a while, but I felt increasingly out of place.

My poker group talked me into playing cards in August. I loved playing poker with the girls. It was well past my turn to host, but I could not even think about that, and they all knew it. My friend Tara was hosting, and she put a special comfortable chair for me at the head of the table. Poker night was fine, but I was very tired and could not eat anything that they served. Tara kept asking me to try this, and I felt like they did not understand why I wasn't eating. I was afraid to eat, and I had no desire to drink wine at this point. I came in second and had an enjoyable time, but little did they know that staying out until 10 pm was huge for me. I was used to going to bed as soon as it got dark.

Overall, my summer was spent battling various gastrointestinal issues, including digestion and nutritional deficiencies, chest tightness of unknown origin, depression, and anxiety. I tried various methods to alleviate my discomfort and pain. I would say that after my phone call with Steve, I improved for a couple of weeks. The heartburn medication was useless. I'm not sure if the acupuncture helped or not, but it was very relaxing. I would give high marks to the infrared sauna therapy. I felt more energized after my sessions. The amino acid IV was probably helpful, but I think I should have done more than one treatment. The digestive enzymes helped me to digest my food when my pancreas was insufficient at doing so. I feel strongly that the EMDR therapy helped me more than my regular sessions. How much of it was depression and anxiety, and how much was actual cell damage from chemo and radiation? I don't know. For me, it felt like one came because of the other. But it did not matter because the stress from depression and anxiety are every bit as harmful to your body!

One day I noticed a post from a woman who was six months post-treatment on my Anal Cancer site, and it read:

OMG!!! I'm stuck in this "pity party," and I can't get out! I'm so sick of being sick and tired: I'm angry and resentful and hating everybody and everything right now. I just want a day when I can eat food, not have to take freaking Imodium or wear a GD diaper! Tried having sex with my husband today. What a joke. There is no way it was fitting in. I know you want to, but don't you dare give me praying hand emojis right now, or I'll lose it for sure!! I'm not even depressed anymore; I'm just pissed off. I HATE cancer and everything that follows it!!

Here are a few of the responses from other members:

I can relate. So over it!

Sat in the car and screamed today! I get it!!

I think the main problem with this Nigro protocol is that 90 some percent of oncologists and radiologists are men while women are increasingly being diagnosed - we all need to be proactive and work towards a new protocol that doesn't destroy your vagina and more! What is new?? This protocol is ancient!!!

Agree!! I researched and found that MD Anderson uses special shields inserted into the vagina before each radiation treatment to protect and preserve the elasticity of the vagina also shielding the cervix. When I asked my male Rad Onc, he dismissed it and said he doesn't use them. Yet, they developed the Hydrogel Space Oars for men with prostate cancer to lessen urinary incontinence and impotence.

Used the recommended dilators faithfully, even tolerated a full-on pap smear. But the skin, omg the skin is like tissue paper. Touch it and it tears and bleeds. Not to mention the nerves or whatever, zero. Nada, felt nothing, couldn't care less.

There is no end to this awful cancer. Been fighting it for two years now.

Yep. I feel like life is passing me by. I think I could handle another type of cancer but this one sucks. Fuck me.

Girl, you know you can vent to me anytime!

Remember the doctors say it's the hardest treatment there is for cancer and the devil's doing his job for sure.

I wish it was any other bloody cancer than this one!!!

Yup!

Agree!

I must have been really bad in a former life to deserve all this shit!!!

Omg!!! Yes. So sorry. Like it hasn't been bad enough, right? Well, put your "big girl" panties on. It's about to get much worse. Please feel free to yell, cry, whine. Whatever you need. We're all here for you and feeling the same shit.

You absolutely deserve a pity party occasionally!

> *It's okay to be feeling this way and we are all here for you. We have all had to lift each other up when we get mad, upset, or depressed. This cancer and this treatment really suck. Someone else already said it but my oncologist said it's the absolute hardest treatment protocol of all the cancers.*

Cry, throw shit, whatever you need to do today. Then tomorrow pick yourself back up.

Thank you. I feel the same way but just did not know how to say it, feel my life is shit and don't know how to get out of this hole, life was great, then the bottom fell out of it. If you find the answer, pass it on.

That sounds horrible. You are a warrior.

We are all warriors; we just have different scars.

"When we think we hurt when we feel we heal.

Adrienne Posey

Chapter 22

Gratitude

I was still trying to gain weight without experiencing gastrointestinal issues. I was warned that this could be a lifelong struggle. I started to maintain my weight which was a step in the right direction. I hovered around 108 to 110 lbs. Mostly my diet consisted of organic steel-cut oats with organic unsweetened fresh or frozen fruit for breakfast, a baked potato or sweet potato or cooked carrots for lunch, lean chicken, or fish with cooked vegetables with lentils or quinoa for dinner. For snacks or dessert, I would have an apple or pear. I was also juicing various vegetables, which unfortunately gave me gas, but I felt it was important for my recovery. I knew that my small bowel and rectum were heavily radiated and were not operating as they should. I was still not absorbing nutrients as I should, and juicing was the best way to achieve that goal.

The tightness in my chest that I experienced was finally getting better. I found out later from others in my Anal Cancer group that Five-FU can indeed cause heart problems. These are serious side effects that do not normally show up on EKGs or in blood tests. It is called dilated cardiomyopathy, and it is when the heart muscle becomes weak and cannot properly pump blood to the rest of the body. I am sure now that this is what I was experiencing. This crushing pain was never heartburn or anxiety. The only way to test for it is with an echocardiogram. I found out later that the infused antimetabolites (chemo drugs) are much more toxic to your heart than those given by bolus. I wish I had known this much earlier. I wish my oncologists would have had this information for me. They should have.

I also knew that the Lexapro was working because my mood improved. I started to want to do things with friends. I went to the movies. I played poker again that month. I rejoined my Saturday golf group. I started to walk my dogs again once a day. I cooked for myself and cleaned up after myself. I exercised a little every day. I continued to see Simone once a week. We did another two sessions of EMDR and then continued our regular sessions. I continued acupuncture on a limited basis. Finally, I finished out my ten pass with Energy Healing. The best thing about September was that it was a turning point for me. I started feeling like I could make plans. I knew that I needed to make plans. Other survivors told me that this was essential. They also told me to be grateful, and I knew I needed to work on that part. So, every night before I went to bed, I would count down ten things I was grateful for. I called it my "gratefulness countdown." Clever, right? I expressed my gratitude for many different things. As an example:

✓ *I am grateful to Ben for helping me so much every day.*

✓ *I am grateful for having enough money to do all these extra alternative treatments.*

✓ *I am grateful for having insurance that covers most of my medical bills.*

✓ *I am grateful for my friends and family who stay connected with me and care about me.*

✓ *I am grateful for my puppies, who make me smile every day.*

✓ *I am grateful to the doctors and nurses who took the time to care for me.*

✓ *I am grateful for all the comforts that my home affords me.*

✓ *I am grateful for all the excellent quality food that I have to eat.*

✓ *I am grateful for the activities that are available near me and for friends that still include me.*

✓ *I am grateful for my health and my recent clear scan.*

I have been told it is important to make plans and to "give back." I planned to write a book and continued journaling my experiences. I planned to start a cancer support group because I could not find one in Prescott for any other cancers except Breast Cancer when I desperately needed one. It's great that they have a Breast Cancer support group, but I felt that I would be out of place there and that we needed one for "all other cancers." I figured I would partner with an oncologist and a naturopath and hold meetings once a month at the library or senior center. I planned to hold a fundraiser someday for the Anal Cancer Foundation. I planned to become a peer-to-peer mentor. I started to sign up for it, but they asked how long since my treatment. They wanted people who were past the two-year mark, so I had to wait. The two-year mark is considered past the danger zone for most recurrences. A person newly diagnosed with Anal Cancer wants to talk to someone who has gone through and survived treatment and is living cancer-free for at least a couple of years or more, if possible. I would need to hold off on giving back right now, but I would be grateful, and I would voice those thanks every night.

My daughter had an event in Las Vegas the second week of September, and I wanted to see her. She invited me to stay in her hotel room and just enjoy what I could for a few days. I decided to make the plan and join her for three nights. It would be a 3.5-hour drive, and Ben was worried, but I felt like I could make the trip without issue.

It was a comfortable room at the south end of the strip, and there was a Starbucks across the street, so I knew where my breakfast would come from. She was involved in the Life Is Beautiful Music Festival in downtown Las Vegas and represented the sponsor, Stella Artois. It was great to see her at work and with her peers. They handled the setup and operation of several marketing promotions that were coinciding with the concert schedule. She did everything from painting backdrops to meeting with city officials for permit issues. I had lunch and dinner with her and ended up leaving just two nights before the start of the festival because she was so busy, and I just felt in the way. I should have just gambled, but I was not really in the mood for it. It was a great trip, but I was glad when I was back home in my own bed.

In July, when I was still in bad shape, a friend from the club referred me to a medical oncologist in Prescott. She was an ER nurse at YRMC hospital, and I valued her opinion. She said that if she were ever to get cancer, she would want no one other than Dr. Hastings to treat her. I called the office in early August, and it took me this long to get an appointment to see him. I wanted to have an oncologist in Prescott for my post-treatment care, and I was so upset with the care I received at Mayo from that department. I had no idea it would take this long to get in to see him. I was not sure after my experience with Dr. Li if I ever wanted to see him again.

I finally met with Dr. Hastings on September 26. Before I contacted his office, I looked up a couple of his reviews online. OMG. One man said that his wife would not be alive today if it were not for Dr. Hastings. Another woman said she hesitated to leave a complimentary review for him because he might get too busy when she needed him. She said he was by far the kindest and most proficient doctor she had ever been to. I figured they were exaggerating. Ben and I walked into his office in Prescott Valley, and it was old but clean. The patients were typical Prescott Valley residents. A man came out of his car and took a seat next to us. His car looked like he was living in it. I tried not to judge. All these people needed oncology care, and I was glad that Prescott and Prescott Valley had a quality oncologist available to treat them. Most good physicians did not stay in Prescott long. They left for the big bucks at the major hospitals.

Dr. Hastings worked out of YRMC north and south in both Prescott and Prescott Valley, and he was affiliated with Arizona Oncology. When Dr. Hastings arrived in the room, we made our introductions. I thanked him for seeing me and told him how highly my friend had spoken of him. I started to rattle off my original diagnosis and treatment at Mayo, and he stopped me and very kindly said that he would like to know more about Bonnie first. I looked up at him and wondered what planet this doctor was from? He had a whole waiting room full of patients waiting to see him, and he was asking me to slow down and talk about myself.

"What do you mean?" I asked.

And he replied, "I mean, tell me about you and your life. Do you have kids, grandkids? Where did you grow up? What brought you to Prescott? Did you or do you work? What do you like to do in your free time? etc...."

So, I told him about myself, and I asked him a few questions too, but he pivoted back to me. Then he asked me how I was feeling now and what my concerns were? I started to tell him about my diagnosis and my scan results, and he stopped me a couple of times and told me that he had reviewed my file and looked at my scans already. I had sent over all my files two months ago, but I was surprised at the length of knowledge he had for my case. Most doctors review a patient's file a few minutes before they walk into the room. This doctor was well-versed in my cancer history, and there was a lot to know. I told him about my visits to the ER, and he knew about those. I told him about the cancer and the chemo agents I received, and he already knew all that.

He wanted to know what problems I was having now, after treatment. I explained the anxiety and depression, then started to cry because he seemed so caring. He handed me the box of tissues and asked me why I was crying. I told him that I was worried about going through all that I had been through and that my cancer would return. He said that we would tackle that together if it ever did, but that right now, I should concentrate on getting stronger. He gave me some ideas on healthy foods that I could eat that would help me to put on weight. He also gave me some added nutritional help. He was a huge fan of lentils and soups and quality proteins. He told me that he was glad that I was on the road to recovery from some of the GI issues and that the rest would get better with time.

He was familiar with the Five FU and Mitomycin and said my labs looked as they should for three months out of treatment. Overall, it was a great visit, and I liked this doctor a lot. I wondered how he could be so patient, take so much time with me, and have such an awesome bedside manner. He was kind and empathetic but also extremely knowledgeable. My friend was right. This was likely the best oncologist in Prescott, and I was lucky to get in to see him. I wished that I had him for my medical oncologist at Mayo. Well, at least I had him now. Hopefully, I would not need him again after today.

I had received an invitation to my friends John and Kyle's wedding, and I was mulling it over. I would be going alone if I went, as Ben didn't want to go to Chicago anymore. I would stay with Michelle and take her as my guest. The wedding was the first weekend in October, and all my old friends from high school and beyond would be attending. I decided to go. It was a great weekend with perfect, crisp but sunny fall weather for their outside wedding. I cried at the ceremony, of course. It was my first gay wedding, and Kyle's daughter from his first marriage gave him away. It touched my heart. Kyle works for an exclusive country club in the north suburbs of Chicago, and he is the Catering Manager. The club provided all the food for the after-party, and I knew that it would be outstanding. Well, it was even better than I expected. I decided to go off my diet and splurge that whole weekend. I got sick, but it was worth it. I saw a lot of friends, and they said how good I looked. I left the wigs at home and wore my hair natural. It was starting to grow in, and I had it trimmed to a super short gray pixie. I think I pulled it off. It was apparent that I was post-chemo, and for the first time in a long time, I felt good about myself. I was just happy to watch as others danced and drank. I sipped on my glass of champagne and enjoyed every minute of it.

I was worried about my bowels on the flight and got aisle seats both ways, just in case. On the way home, a lady much younger than me asked me if I would not mind letting her have the aisle seat because she had an issue with her bladder, and she was carrying a cane and walked with a heavy limp. I told her that it was fine. I did not have the heart or desire to argue with her about my own problems. I was worried the whole time about going in an emergency and having to ask her, of all people, to get up for me. Would she be able to get up quickly for me? I made it the four hours, and the issues were moot, but it made me realize that I was not the only person with health problems on that plane. I don't know who had things worse, but it didn't matter. We were both in the same boat or plane rather.

My friend Amy is a member of a different club called Capital Canyon. Amy is a close friend who has gone out of her way to help me with my home and dogs while I was in treatment. Her husband died of cancer, and she knows first-hand what it's like to be a caregiver and how toxic the treatments can be to patients. She asked me to play in her Member-Guest Tournament, and she would not let me pay a dime toward the entry fee. I was not sure yet about playing two days in a row, but I felt like I could take a stab at it. As is customary when playing with Amy, we dressed to match. She has a sewing machine and offered to take in one of my outfits that matched hers.

Had we not taken it in, it would have fallen right off me. She took it in a full four inches on both the top and bottom. We looked great with matching fuchsia and white-flowered golf outfits. Amy even brought me a pair of socks to match on the morning of our first day. Each morning of the two-day tournament, we had a breakfast buffet served outside on the practice range. The weather was great, and several ladies came up to me to say how nice it was to see me out playing golf again. I made it through the entire tournament and attended the dinner afterward. I put on my wig for the dinner and wore a new outfit that I purchased (size 2). I had a glass of champagne that I sipped on most of the afternoon. I even tried a couple of the appetizers. I chose a salmon dish for my entree and ate nearly all of it. We didn't win anything, but I felt like a winner for just showing up.

A few of the small-framed ladies at my club got word that I was golfing again and decided to clean out their closets and dropped off piles of golf outfits for me. I was very appreciative. I, in turn, took my size 10 and 12 clothes to the club and offered them up to anyone interested. It felt like I had a whole new wardrobe. We should do this when we get tired of our clothes, too, because one woman's clutter could well be another woman's treasure.

I played in another one-day event at our club a couple of weeks later, and my partner and I came in first place for our net score. I played fine, and she played great, making every putt in sight. It was great to compete again. Even though I only helped on a few holes, I still helped. I played another round of golf with friends at our nearby public course, and we went for drinks and appetizers after. Ben and I took a short weekend trip to Tucson with Amy and Tim, and all went well. I was getting stronger and feeling better. Of course, there were days that I had GI issues, but I was learning to control those issues with my diet. At the end of October, I went to Seattle to visit Fran. She has a Halloween party every year, so I even dressed up and helped her shop, cook, and clean. I wasn't sure that travel would be something that I could do post-treatment again, but it looks like I will be able to retain that freedom. I felt incredibly grateful for that.

In November, I stopped seeing Simone and went off the Lexapro. I was worried that my depression would return, but it did not. I also stopped going to the acupuncturist and finished a ten pack at Energy Health and Wellness. With my clear scan and mental health back on track, I decided to switch my focus to cancer prevention. I made follow-up appointments with Dr. Zander and Dr. Rubin because I finally felt well enough to start up a full prevention plan. While working on my mental health, I realized that worrying about the future was still causing me a great deal of stress. I did not want my cancer to return, and I could take rational steps to prevent that.

Along with several supplements, they both strongly suggested high-dose vitamin C three times per week. Dr. Zander thought it was important to add IV Artesunate. Arsenate is an isolate from the plant Artemisia annua L. (Sweet wormwood). Dr. Zander told me that it is an anti-angiogenic (meaning it helped prevent tumors from making new blood vessels and worked synergistically with the vitamin C.) Recent studies showed it improved survival in stage 4 Breast Cancer patients and that there was growing evidence that it worked in other cancers as well. I decided to add the artesunate to my arsenal even though Dr. Rubin was not convinced it would help that much. Dr. Rubin was a big proponent of IV quercetin.

Quercetin can be found in many foods such as apples, honey, and onions. It acts as an antioxidant just like vitamin C. Recent studies in vivo and in vitro show that this flavonoid complex can induce apoptosis and prevent cancer cell lines in many types of cancers. It is also anti-viral and anti-inflammatory. After much research, I decided to add it to my arsenal. I could not find a source for it in Prescott, so I decided to go to Dr. Rubin's office once a week for my infusions. Quercetin had a short shelf life and had to be ordered from a compounding pharmacy that delivered one time per week. It was not only hard to obtain, but it was costly as well. The IV bag was huge and took more than two and a half hours to infuse.

Dr. Rubin also suggested a medication that was just recently approved for use in the US. It was being used with superior results in Europe. Thymosin Alpha 1 (1500 mcg 2 x weekly per SQ injection) is a hormone that contains 28 amino acids. It is an immunotherapy agent, and she sent me some literature on it. I researched it as best I could. It was all overly complicated, and I must admit, I was putting a lot of faith in Dr. Rubin. My concern was that it was a pharmaceutical and therefore could have strong side effects. It had been studied in several different cancers, but nothing was ever studied in my type of cancer because it was so rare and did not elicit the funds necessary for clinical trials. The studies showed remarkable effects. This drug could stimulate my immune system and make it work better. I added it to my arsenal. It came from a pharmacy somewhere in Utah, and it had to be kept refrigerated. Like my mistletoe injections, I began to inject it into my stomach two times per week.

Zander wanted me to take a much stronger Mistletoe dose, and he said that I could add it to my Vitamin C IV. I was happy about this because it was much easier than injecting it. The Viscum Albus 100 was now being added to every Vitamin C infusion.

My newest protocol was underway. I had to cut back on my golf schedule, but I was determined. I had a scan coming up, and I wanted it to be clear. I spent most of my weekdays sitting in either Dr. Rubin's or Dr. Zander's office. When you go in for an infusion, you first meet with the nurse who accesses your vein and inserts the catheter. From there, you are hooked up to the bag of nutrients, and you sit. I would bring my laptop or reading materials. Sometimes I would just catch up on calls or texts. If I was tired, I would sleep. I never made it through the entire bag without a trip to the lady's room. That was always a chore. I had to bring my pole and bag with me and make sure I did not kink the line or bend my arm too much. I made effective use of my time, and it passed quickly.

In early December, the PLWGA (Prescott Lakes Women's Golf Association) had its annual Christmas Luncheon. I decided to attend since it would be a wonderful place to catch up with many of the ladies I had not seen in months and thank them personally for their cards and gifts. I was a board member for the last two years and used to oversee planning this party. We celebrated the holiday, and it acted as our end-of-the-year board meeting where we recognized special achievements and tournament winners. This year, I was supposed to act again as the Tournament Chair, but I had to turn it over to another after my diagnosis. In addition to the Christmas Luncheon, the Tournament Chair was also in charge of four yearly tournaments that the PLWGA sponsored. Our PLWGA held a Spring Kickoff, a Charity Tournament, a Fall Partners Event, and a Member-Guest Event. The Tournament Chair position could be challenging. I was in charge of recruiting people to run the tournaments and overseeing them in their respective roles. It was always difficult to find members to step up and volunteer to run a tournament, so I ran a couple of tournaments myself over the years.

The first year, I ran the Spring Kick-off, and we did a Chicago theme. It was a hoot. Unfortunately, the weather was windy and cold that day, but it fit the theme! I enjoyed event planning, so it was fun for me. I put a lot of work into my tournaments, and everything had to fit the theme. For our Chicago Tournament, we entertained on the staging area with songs from Chicago artists only. I formed a committee of several volunteers. Of course, they all had to be from Chicago or Illinois originally. We dressed up in various sports team attire (Cubs, Bulls, Bears, and Blackhawks) and performed a little skit. We also had a separate skills contest on the Putting Green where we named the puts after Chicago landmarks. The decor was all Black and Red, and when you walked into the clubhouse, we had a cow kicking over a lantern with tissue paper flames. I could not get deep-dish pizza, so we had an Italian lunch and had our pro dress up as a mobster and come in with a toy machine gun during lunch. Our big show was when our whole committee dressed up as the Blues Sisters, dancing and singing to *Sweet Home Chicago*.

I also headed up the 3-day Member-Guest Tournament for the last two years. Our theme was "Age of Aquarius" in 2017, and it was such a hit, I decided to do it again in 2018. The Member-Guest is when you invite another lady from outside of the club. Some brought their moms or daughters or invited friends from out of town. Some got gals from neighboring clubs. It was a hoot. We had flowers everywhere and painted pet rocks for everyone. Our gifts were hippie bags and mandala scarves. Our pre-party was a full 60's and 70's bash with hors d'oeuvres from that era. We burned incense and made flower headbands for all the women. We had fire dancers and served Jiffy Pop after dark. For lunch, we served food from that era. One year we made up TV dinners in foil trays with cardboard tops. We even had a big wooden magic bus as a photo backdrop. Most of the women dressed up in matching hippie attire.

I planned to do the Member-Guest Tournament again in 2019 and do a Viva Las Vegas theme. I even started looking into booking an Elvis Impersonator, but … life had other plans for me. I missed the entire year of what used to be a big part of my life. Oh well, I was determined to make the most of this new challenge. I now considered it an opportunity to work on myself. What else could I do? I had no choice.

Several years back, one member made a huge pair of satin panties, and I mean huge! She made them for a member who had gone through some difficulties that year. She presented them to her at the Christmas luncheon. "Put on your big girl panties and get through it." That was the idea behind the Big Girl Panties. From that time, each year, the panties are presented to another member. There were suspenders added so that they could be worn for a photograph. Well, as you can imagine, they were presented to me in 2019, so I proudly wore them for the photograph and hung them on my tree out in front of my house for a couple of weeks before Christmas. Everyone said how happy they were to see me back out again and that I looked good. I was glad that I went even though I could not eat the food served or drink liquor.

I did not have the energy or time to decorate the outside of our house, but Ben decided to step up and take charge of that. Carli, Sean, and the grandkids would be coming in for about five nights starting on Dec 25. We had an enjoyable time, and I did my best to join in their activities, but the food was always an issue for me. Like most young families in this country, they loved to eat out, and mostly it consisted of highly processed and fast food that contained an overabundance of sugar and fat. I often found myself eating separately from the rest of them. I had given up long ago trying to convince them to make better choices. I did not want to be that person who thinks they know better. Now I had even less credibility. *Who is the one who got cancer?*

Unfortunately, my cancer, unlike some others, had little to do with a poor diet. A virus caused it, but no matter the cause, diet was a crucial factor in having a strong immune system. Now more than ever, I was a huge proponent of improving one's immune system to fight all kinds of diseases, including cancer. Carli was probably the best mother I knew, but she had no idea why her children got so many colds and ear infections every year. It was obvious that it had a lot to do with their diets and an over-dependence on antibiotics. They were young and still had strong immune systems, but I knew all too well that their immune systems would start to decline with age, and good, early habits would be worth their weight in gold someday. But who was I to preach, especially now?

Our family left right before New Year's Eve. We had gotten an invite from Amy to join them at Capital Canyon for their New Year's Eve party. This year's theme was Casino Royale. I convinced Ben to go. He hated dressing up, and due to the theme, it was formal attire. He wore a suit and borrowed a peacock feather bow tie from a friend. He looked great. I shopped for dresses with Amy and found a skin-tight one. It was a bit too sexy, so she took in a dress that I had previously worn. It was gold and black and full of sequins and was perfect for the occasion. Many of the ladies, including Amy, wore full-length gowns. It was a fun event with lots of dancing and gambling. I gambled but did not dance. I was never a great dancer, and now I had a good excuse. We celebrated with the east coast at ten pm since we are an old crowd and were home by eleven. I stayed up until midnight and made a resolution for 2020. I never made a resolution before in my life. It just wasn't my thing. This year, I decided I would try to change. I wanted to live my life to its fullest and make a difference in the lives of others. I made a promise to be a better listener and to be more empathetic to others. This was something specific that I could do to be a better person. After all the months I spent reflecting on my life, I realized that I was probably a poor listener. It's not that I did not care about what others were saying. It is more about my wanting or needing to be liked. I often caught myself thinking of what I would say next, and then I missed out on what others were saying.

This did not happen with my old friends because I was comfortable with them. It happened with new acquaintances. It happened with people I was trying too hard to impress. I know it's a common personality trait, but I wanted to change it in me. I knew that when I was hurting, some people were good listeners and others were not. Those good listeners were a tremendous help to me, and I wanted to be one of them. I wanted to care more about others and care less about what they thought of me. Cancer had changed me, and this resolution did not take much effort on my part. I looked at life much differently now. I no longer cared as much about what others thought of me. When people complained about their lives, I would listen and be kind. I would not offer advice unless they asked for it. Life is not a popularity contest. Even when they complained about trivialities, I would try to understand where they were coming from and what may have shaped them to act this way. We have all had diverse backgrounds and experiences, and I had no right to judge.

"There is a club in this world that you do not join knowingly. One day you are just a member. It is 'The life-changing events club.' The fee to join is hurt beyond belief, payable in full, upfront for a lifetime membership. The benefit of the club is a newfound perspective on life and a deep understanding that you may not be happy about your current situation, but you can be happy in your current situation. The only rule to the club is that you cannot tell anyone that you are a member. The club does not provide a directory of its members, but when you look into a member's eye, you can tell that they, too, are part of the club. Members are allowed to exchange that brief eye contact that says: 'I didn't know.' Being a member of this club is the last thing that anyone initially wants in their life. Being a member of this club is the best thing that ever happens to a person in their life, and there is not a person in the club that would ever give up their membership. If you really look and know what you are looking for, you can spot the club's members; they are the ones that provide a random act of kindness and do something for someone who can never repay them for what they have done. They are the people spreading joy and optimism and lifting people's spirits even when their own heart has been broken. I have paid my dues; my lifetime membership arrived today, not by mail, but by a deep inner feeling that I cannot describe. It is the best club that I never wanted to be part of. But I am glad that I am a member."

John Passaro

Part 2

Levity

Chapter 23

Acceptance

My days were filled with juicing, taking my supplements, giving myself subcutaneous injections, and infusions of Vitamin C, Artesunate, Mistletoe, and Quercetin. I continued expressing my gratitude nightly for all I had in my life and for having survived this setback. I golfed occasionally and worked on my book. Our friends were busy planning their winter vacations to get away from the cold. Amy and Tim asked us to join them in Cabo, but I could not. I had scans coming up and did not feel comfortable traveling with friends yet. I was starting to get some short waves of anxiety over my upcoming scans. I knew that I was now doing everything I could to stop the cancer from coming back, but I also knew deep down that I had wasted several months of precious time when I was too sick to work on my immune system.

We started hearing in the news about a new virus that had begun in China. It was very surreal to see people wearing masks on the news. It felt like a science fiction movie, but it was real. We talked about it with our friends and family, but like most things that happen on the other side of the planet, such as wars, famine and the like, we felt it was isolated to that area and that we were protected by distance. How wrong I would be about that.

I was golfing two days a week now. I played on Tuesdays and Saturdays. In many ways, I was getting stronger every day and starting to enjoy competing again, with my new higher handicap, of course. I began to swing the club with more confidence, and with that new swing, I developed a nagging pain in my lower back. I was overdoing it. That must be it. Then it started bothering me when I walked the dogs. I must have pulled a muscle. I started to cut back on golfing again, and I iced and put heat on my back. It was not unusual for me to have lower back issues. I had a problem in the past with my SI joint. It got inflamed now and then, and I simply needed to rest it. It never bothered me when I walked before. This was a bit concerning. Even though I was cutting back on my golf, the pain gradually increased, so I decided it had to be from my rebounding. I would jump on the rebounder 900 times per day. It was part of my exercise routine. I decided to stop the jumping, and it still got worse. I started having to rest halfway through my walks with the dogs. I just sat on the ground or the curb, and after a short rest, I was fine. It was weird. This was different than the back pain I had in the past.

In February of 2020, the news of the Virus started becoming more of a concern. It was now in several areas of Asia. There was talk that it started from bats and that those bats may have bitten domestic animals sold for human consumption at one of the markets in China. Now it was becoming widespread in Asia, and there were reports of the virus spreading to Europe. We had one confirmed case in the US. China and North Korea were now in full lockdown. We live in a global economy, so I wondered how we would stop this virus from coming into the states. It was just a matter of time.

On February 26, I was scheduled for my scans. We headed down to Mayo, where I first went for my labs. I then headed to the lower level of building three for my CT scan. I was getting a picture of my chest, abdomen, and pelvis. It was nerve-wracking as usual. I knew that if the cancer came back, it would do so in the first year or two. After the scans were done, we went for a bite to eat and returned to Dr. Jordan's office for the results. He started out by telling me that my blood tests looked good. My absolute Lymphocytes were still extremely low, but he said that overall, my white counts looked good. Then I looked into his eyes, and I saw the look.

"It's not good, right?" I asked. The CT scan was not good. I could tell before he spoke.

He said, "We have some concerning spots in your lungs that were not there on the last scan. Unfortunately, it's too small to know for sure what it is, and many things are floating in the air in Arizona."

"Could it be inflammation," I asked, hoping for the best.

"It is possible you breathed something into your lungs that irritated it," he replied. "It could be inflammation and nothing to be concerned about. But unfortunately, we can't rule out metastasis."

Glancing at the radiology report, it was right there: "Possible metastasis."

"We need to schedule another test in three months to see if there is any change with the spots. It is too small even to do a PET scan yet. All we can do is wait," said Dr. Jordan.

Curiously, I was not that upset. Somewhere deep in my subconscious, I knew this day would come. I had prepared myself for it, and I knew that there was plenty that I could do besides WAIT! I was not going to sit back and do nothing.

It was another quiet ride home. We talked about how the spots could be something else and let it go at that. My mind started to drift to a darker place, and I began to question why I could never catch a break. Why did I keep getting bad news? Why couldn't I be like the other survivors in my Facebook group who went right back to work after treatment and lived cancer-free for years now? Then I stopped myself and thought about others who had to have APR (abdominoperineal resection) surgery because their initial treatment did not work. At least I did not need a colostomy. I also thought about those patients who died during treatment. I was still alive, and I had a decent quality of life. I knew that if this were a metastasis, I would now be technically a stage 4, but stage 4 or not, I HAD to stop feeling sorry for myself!!!!

In March, the Coronavirus started to spread rampantly through Europe. I never thought I would see something like this in my life. People started wearing masks, and Trump was now doing a daily press briefing with Dr. Fauci and Dr. Birx as his task force. Dr. Anthony Fauci is the Director of the National Institute of Allergy and Infectious Diseases, and Dr. Birx was hired as our Coronavirus Response Coordinator. They said that if we did things perfectly from now on out, we could still expect up to 200,000 US deaths, and if we did nothing to control it, we could expect as many as 2.2 million. We began to wear masks in public and to disinfect everything that we brought into our homes. Strange times for sure!

The individual states started to close certain types of businesses like bars, gyms, and movie theaters. Events were being canceled everywhere. People were losing their jobs, and new guidelines were implemented to limit the virus from spreading. There were more restrictions on airline travel as well. Trump started to worry about the economy and for his chances for reelection. The economy was his strongest achievement. His daily press briefings got weird. Fauci and Birx would say one thing, and then he would say another. For example, they would suggest that all people wear masks and socially distance, and Trump would say it's up to the individual and praise the states that kept their businesses open. Trump would never wear a mask in public, so many of his supporters embraced that same lack of respect. Politics entered heavily into the handling of the Virus, and what a mistake that was! By the end of March, cases were soaring. It seemed curious to me that my life was now being controlled by two very distinct but equally deadly viruses.

"No matter what happens during any given day, I know I have a higher power to call on; this vast universe to create with, and the sublime knowledge that there is always a way to rise up even when there doesn't seem to be a way out."

Anonymous

Chapter 24

Clarity

So, the odds, according to my oncologists, are that my cancer has metastasized. If it turns out to be inflammation, that will be fantastic, but I must take this seriously. I have just three months to see if I can make a difference. Is it a different protocol now that it's metastatic (in my blood)? I must see Dr. Rubin and Dr. Zander again to find out. I make those appointments, and due to Covid, they will be by Telemed. That's fine with me. I'm in no hurry to catch this deadly virus. I can get a quicker appointment this way. My days will now be completely dedicated to stopping or reversing the growth of my cancer. I start to become most uncomfortable with the word cancer. I am using it nonstop, and it has such a negative connotation to it. I decide to start calling it by another name. After much deliberation, I decide on UG. It stands for Uncontrolled Growth. That means that all that is necessary is to control it. We are so anxious to kill it, that we cut it out, poison ourselves systemically or burn our tumors and any areas of spread. It is barbaric. Perhaps, all we need to do is to control it.

Look at Aids. People used to think of Aids as the kiss of death, but now people simply live with it. It is controlled. When someone is diagnosed with UG, their first thought is usually "get this out of me now." If you think about it, that makes no sense. It's often not something we can just cut, burn, or poison out of us immediately. It can be systemic, and even if they get all of the tumor, the stem cells often remain. It takes a long time for most UGs to grow, and therefore we should not expect to rid our bodies of it in one fell swoop and at any cost. By calling it Uncontrolled Growth, I am reserving my right to simply control and weaken it to a point where it can be successfully destroyed and hopefully by my very own immune system. If it is not causing me any pain, maybe I can just keep it small and live with it. The bottom line, once we figure out how to harness and support our immune systems to fight against this invader, we can stop fearing UG.

I began my thirst for knowledge on the subject and read as many books as possible. I also joined many Facebook groups in a quest to speak to as many survivors as possible to find out what steps they took to control or reverse their UGs. I learned that a viral UG was just like any other and could be weakened. I needed to stop feeding it. More accurately, I needed to stop fueling it. Now I know the environment that UG thrives in. It likes an acidic environment, and therefore, I needed my body to be as alkaline as possible. It feeds on glucose, and all carbs will convert to glucose, so I need to go on a very low-carb diet. The UG cells have low oxygen levels, and these low oxygen levels have proven to be a key driver in many types of UGS. They thrive in an anaerobic state. I need to get oxygen to my cells.

Much of UG research thus far has centered around genetic mutations, but now there is growing evidence that when an UG cell gets more food, it grows and becomes more hypoxic (without enough oxygen). It can hide from our immune systems and mimic normal cells. It can create its own blood vessels. Researchers are discovering that chemotherapeutic agents work for a while and then stop working because this oxygen and fueling issue is never resolved. To control or reverse UG by limiting its fueling capacities is known as the Metabolic Approach. To me, it makes sense to attack UG from every angle, especially when it is systemic or when organs are involved. I am not completely against surgery, chemo, and radiation. I just believe that we can and should do more metabolic research and treatments.

This is what I can do for myself now. I can exercise more. This will increase the oxygen in my blood and keep my heart strong. I can keep my stress level down; stress is a killer. I will achieve this through mindfulness and meditation. I will stay in the present. I can't look back, and I won't look forward because I am not a psychic. I must connect spiritually somehow. Every survivor of advanced UG that I spoke with gave me this same advice. They all had a strong spiritual connection of some sort, and they remained positive because of it. Lastly, I would enhance my immune system and stop fueling my UG. I already knew a lot about enhancing my immune system, but how exactly would I stop fueling my UG. It was an overly complicated subject. Hopefully, Dr. Rubin and Dr. Zander could help me with that.

After my Saturday round of golf, I was getting shooting pains and numbness down my legs. It was getting worse instead of better. I decided it would be best to give myself a complete rest from golf. I was feeling it now every time I walked the dogs. I would get about halfway through my walk, and the pain in my legs would get so bad that I had to sit down and rest. I chalked it up to my sciatic nerve.

My call with Dr. Zander came first, and he was devastated to hear the news. I told him that it was not definite, but his voice told me otherwise. He scheduled more blood work for me, and we discussed how to handle this best. He wanted me to continue with my high-dose vitamin C and artesunate. He also wanted me to increase my dosage of mistletoe to 100 mg. That was five times what I was currently taking! I asked about ozone treatments to address the oxygen issue, and he agreed this would be a good idea if I could afford it. We talked about several other supplements, and I was honest with him about my upcoming consultation with Dr. Rubin. I wanted both of their perspectives. When I mentioned my leg pain to Dr. Zander, he seemed concerned about the possibility of enlarged lymph nodes pressing on a nerve. This concerned me as well. I told him that I would call Dr. Jordan to get his opinion. We scheduled a follow-up after my blood test results came in.

I had an appointment coming up with Dr. Hastings, so I brought it up to him. He said he doubted that my lymph nodes could cause that problem, but he did not rule it out. He looked over my recent scan and agreed with the wait and rescan approach. We discussed my GI issues, and I told him that my heartburn was finally better. I stopped taking the Prilosec and was only on the Lexapro now. He recommended that I stay on it for a few more months. He also recommended alternating ice and heat on my back.

My call with Dr. Rubin went well. He was also disappointed in my scan. He was hoping our protocol would prevent this. He wanted to shift focus on a few of our strategies now that it could be systemic. He took me off the Thymosin Alpha. He figured that it was not working. Where Dr. Rubin and Dr. Zander disagreed, most was on the use of mistletoe right now. Dr. Rubin said that he would not order it for me during Covid. Dr. Zander insisted that it was important. He also worried about me taking the AHCC mushroom complex during Covid, and I didn't understand why. We talked about Covid a lot. Dr. Rubin was just as concerned about keeping me safe from Covid as he was about keeping me safe from my UG. I didn't feel the same way. He kept me on Naltrexone and suggested a new RX called TM or Tetra Thiomolybdate. which was some type of copper chelator. I didn't understand it and said that I would look into it. If I went on it, I would need to keep an eye on my liver enzymes with regular blood testing. I would also need to test my CBC and ceruloplasmin after two weeks. I would start with a low dose and increase it to the optimum tolerable dose. He could tell that I was getting overwhelmed, so he said that he would send me literature on its benefits. We added 20 mg of Melatonin nightly, Pectasol C (5 grams 2 X daily 10-12 hours apart), Berberine (500 mg daily for one week then increase to 500mg 2x daily 10-12 hours apart, then after one week, I would increase it to 1000mg in the AM and 500 mg in the PM). We also added Quercisorb-SR (2capsules daily, Transresveratrol (1000 mg 2 x daily, Black Cumin Seed Oil (2 capsules 2 x daily with food), Cura Pro (1 gel cap 1X daily with food), Zinc Bisglycinate (54 mg 2 x daily with food), Long Vida (400 mg 1 x daily), Turiva (1 x daily) and Curcumin (800 mg 1 x daily). Holy cow, I thought. As for the IV treatments, he suggested 4000 mcg of ozone for my first treatment and increased to 70,000 on my second, third, and then weekly. He said that the Vitamin C would be hard to find now with Covid but that I needed it a minimum of three times a week. I would also continue with the Quercetin at least once per week (although he recommended 2x). For Covid protection, he wanted me on 400 mg of CoQ10, 300 mg of Super Strength Coriolis, 1t C-RLA 2 x daily, and three drops of Bio D Mulsion Forte (D3).

These new protocols from Dr. Zander and Dr. Rubin were beyond overwhelming. Some people might think they were taking advantage of me, but I knew this was not the case. They believed that they could help me, and I knew that many others like me benefited from these same supplements and protocols. I heard it repeatedly. We shared our protocols on Facebook with one another and let others know what was working for us and what was not. UG patients were extending their lives and sometimes curing their own UGs with just these therapies alone. Some of them turned down surgery, chemo, and radiation and did only integrative or naturopathic. Some of them did both. Most of them have been through conventional treatments and have been told they can no longer be helped.

We never judged. I read a book called 'Radical Remission' by Kelly Turner, Ph.D. Turner, a researcher, lecturer, and counselor in Integrative Oncology. She was shocked to learn that no one was studying radical remissions in people who have recovered against all odds. So, she spent eight years traveling the world searching for once terminal patients who are now surviving and thriving. Here is a list of the nine things that they all have in common:

- ✓ Radically changed their diets
- ✓ Deepened their spiritual connections
- ✓ Increased positive emotions
- ✓ Released suppressed emotions
- ✓ Taking herbs and vitamins
- ✓ Use intuition to help make health decisions
- ✓ Took control of their own health
- ✓ Have strong reasons to live
- ✓ Receiving social support

I kept calm about my possible metastasis. My schedule was hectic, so I had no time to dwell on it. I did all my Vitamin C, artesunate, and mistletoe at Dr. Zander's office. I also did my ozone (03) treatments there as they were considerably cheaper than what Dr. Rubin offered. Unfortunately, we did them the old-fashioned way and did not use Dr. Rubin's fancy ten-pass machine. I hoped that it would work just as well and be safe. I had heard from others that it could cause an embolism or blood clot if not done properly. I believe this is how Farah Fawcett died. That didn't stop me.

Once a week, I went in, and the nurse put in an IV and removed a bag of blood. The bag had to be lower than my arm so that it drained out of me. I must admit that I was a bit tentative about the procedure the first time, but I got used to it after a while. Then she took the bag and added ozone with a large syringe to my blood. She turned the bag a few times to mix it in, and I got it put back in by drip. It obviously took a lot longer going back in than it did coming out. Although ozone therapy is used as a standard UG treatment in many parts of the world, the US considers it an alternative, and most people's insurance will not cover it. The first time I did my 100mg of mistletoe, I went shopping the next day and noticed that I had a lump in my stomach about the size of a golf ball. I panicked because my first thought was that it was a tumor. Then I remembered that this was the exact spot where I administered my mistletoe. That was a huge relief. I knew it meant that the mistletoe was doing what it was supposed to do. I recalled that I would get a tiny bump when I took the smaller doses in the past, so the big golf ball made sense, now that I have increased the dosage so dramatically.

I continued my visits to the infrared sauna. Some weeks I went as many as five times. I figured that I might as well get my money's worth, and I loved how it made me feel. This is also where I listened to many of my audible books. I elevated a book titled "Immune System Booster Affirmations" by Stevens Hyang to the top of my list. It is not a book but more of an audible hypnosis therapy, better known as healing meditation through repetitive affirmations. Self-hypnosis is achieved through the calm music and the soothing narrator's voice. I made myself as comfortable as possible, and I tried to visualize and embrace each affirmation. I considered the phrases in the most positive way.

I would often imagine a force of tiny soldiers as I repeated the narrator's gentle voice. "I am the healthiest I can be." "I allow my body to transform into its best version." "I let my mind determine my health." "I can strengthen my immune system with my mind." "My mind is focused on strengthening my immune system." "I can attain perfect health no matter what." "I am perfectly in tune with my body." "Every pain is my body's message to me." I feel happy and grateful for just being alive." "I am impressed by my immune system." "I am in awe of how my immune system functions." "I send love to every cell of my body." "I am responsible for my health." "I am strong." "My body's immune system gets stronger with each breath I take." "My body is resilient." "My immune system is a genius." "I am brimming with vitality." "I am thankful for my body's natural ability to heal." "I am healing from all the disease I have." "I receive powerful healing energy from the infinite source." "I am full of positive energy."

I already believed strongly in the mind/body connection, so this would only strengthen that belief. When I closed my eyes, I envisioned that brigade of soldiers with tiny helmets on. They were marching through my lymph system and around my diseased cells. They busied themselves scraping off and collecting the debris that was toxic to my body. The smallest particles were hosed down, and the larger pieces were put into tiny wheelbarrows and wheeled down to my liver for detoxification. I envisioned myself sweating out the small particles through my pores. After my session, I showered off the sweat and felt like a cleansing had just taken place. All of this happened simply with the power of my mind. When your immune system is depressed, it might just need a big hug!

The rescan went smoothly at Mayo, and as usual, I braced myself for the results. With a bewildered look, Dr. Jordan tells me that the spots on my lungs are now gone. I am elated. Then he delivers the bad news. The lymph nodes deep in my stomach are now enlarged. He called them my para-aortic nodes. It looked to him like three to five nodes were involved. I remained calm. I processed his statement in a clear and objective way. I asked if he thought it could just be inflammation. In my mind, I imagined that they could be inflamed if they were eliminating toxins from my body. It made perfect sense to me since the lymph is the body's drainage system. He said that it was possible but was concerning because my UG is known to spread there. He seemed apologetic about not seeing their involvement prior to my treatment, and he said that we could still radiate them if necessary. This was not something that I wanted to hear.

Of course, I was not angry with him for not catching what might have been microscopic last year. I asked how big they were, and he told me that the largest one measured 1.5 cm on the large side. I then told him about my back and leg pain, and he said that he thought they were too small to cause something like that but that he would refer me to Dr. Janek in PT for further evaluation. We made that call immediately, and she could squeeze me in that same day for a quick exam to figure out where my pain might be originating. Dr. Jordan said that the next step would be a PET scan which would confirm the diagnosis. I asked if there was any other way to determine if this was for sure UG, and he said that it would be a bad area to try and get a needle biopsy from, but if I wanted to look into that, he could do some further testing. I told him that I would not be interested in a biopsy. I did not want them to open up anything that was contained. He wanted to set up the PET scan as soon as possible. I reluctantly told him to go ahead, even though I knew that it meant injecting more glucose into my body to feed any spots of UG!

I remained optimistic about the lymph nodes being just inflammation. The spots on my lungs went away. I was beginning to realize that diagnosing UG was not an exact science, especially without a biopsy. Radiologists can see only so much from a CT scan. They can't tell the difference between inflammation and UG. The PET scan is then used to make the confirmation. At the same time, waiting for my next appointment with PT, I looked up some statistics on the efficacy of CT and PET scans in UG diagnoses. OMG! They are not that accurate. A CT scan has the potential to be completely wrong in 30% of cases. A PET or Positron Emission Tomography is more definitive, but for some UGS, it is not that useful, especially when the tumor is small. Overall, the combination of both tests is about 75% accurate. That statistic comes from the National Cancer Institute at the National Institute of Health. I thought about how many people might have been treated for UG unnecessarily, especially in the past when scans were much less accurate than today.

During my exam with Dr. Janek, she asked me to stand and lay in certain positions, and she pressed on my bones and soft tissue, mostly around my hip area. She left the room and came back with a diagnosis that my pain was from those para-aortic lymph nodes. She looked at my scans and called her husband, a medical oncologist, for his opinion. I was disappointed in that conclusion.

My PET scan was scheduled for next week. I wasn't the type to sit around and wait, so I made a follow-up appointment with Dr. Zander. He told me to go out and get some castor oil and sheets of wool and follow the directions for a castor oil pack. He admitted that it sounded silly, but he said it works to help drain lymph nodes. You soak the sham with the oil, heat it up in the microwave, and apply it to the affected area. He told me to do this every night. Almost 90% of the fatty acid in castor oil is something called Ricinoleic Acid. Research shows that it effectively prevents the growth of numerous species of viruses, bacteria, yeasts, and molds. Castor Oil also helps improve the flow and movement of lymph fluid through the vessels. Dr. Zander also suggested a few other changes but mostly to keep doing what I was doing because obviously some things were working or were in the process of working. I saw that logic as clear as day, but I was not quite ready to completely dismiss the expert knowledge of the doctors at Mayo. It made sense that my nodes were causing my back and leg pain, and my own research confirmed that Dr. Jordan was right about my anal UG liking to go to those particular lymph nodes. As your lymph system goes, it is not governed by the laws of gravity. The lymph system drains upward and outward in the body.

While waiting for my PET scan results, I felt some trepidation. I was hoping that I could handle whatever was thrown at me. Dr. Jordan got right to the point and showed me a few nodes that lit up to an SUV of 13.4 and a few others around 8.5. They were in my para-aortic area. I also had other areas that were concerning in my lungs and upper chest. He said that UG is highly active when presented with glucose, and I knew this to be true. I asked if anything else could cause this, and he said that some things might cause a slight uptake value, but he felt that the nodes in the back of my stomach were definitely UG. He also felt that the others in my lungs were highly suspect. He looked at me and waited for my reaction. I had none; I was apathetic. I was sad, and Ben was too, but we processed the news. I pulled up my big girl panties. So be it; I was not done with this fight. Not by any sense of the word. Stage 4 was just a number. I knew plenty of others that were living with Stage 4, and I could do it too.

Dr. Jordan said that he spoke with Dr. Li, and they agreed that the chemotherapy did not do its job. It was supposed to mop up whatever radiation did not kill. I then felt angry that I did it for nothing. I did not blame them. My doctors were only doing the best that they could with the training and knowledge that they had. They only had certain treatments available to prescribe for me. I thought about how the pharmaceutical companies owned and funded medical schools and how that seemed so unethical. I know that chemotherapy kills a lot of UG patients. I'm pretty sure that it damaged my heart. It could have killed me, and for what? I asked what they recommended as a next step, and Jordan said they could now put me on the Opdivo. *Really???* I thought to myself. *Now they can give it to me?* I was trying so hard to get it BEFORE my treatment, and now that I am stage 4, they can offer it to me. He said that because the chemotherapy did not work, they could convince my insurance company to allow it off-label. Dr. Jordan then admitted that his first thought was to radiate the nodes and that Dr. Li convinced him that immunotherapy was in my better interest since the UG was metastatic. Thank you, Dr. Li. Why would he want to radiate my nodes if the UG was in several areas? Was he going just to keep zapping me when they popped up? This is what they would do if immunotherapy were not available. This is what patients went through and still go through in many small-town hospitals. Each time it grows or pops up in a new location, they radiate, surgically remove it, or try a new chemotherapy agent. Most stubborn UGS don't respond to chemo because not only does it rarely kill the stem cells, but it often mutates and adapts. Therefore, chemo can work at first and then stop working. It's not a fair fight. I know it. They know it too. Yet, they keep giving it to their patients. Whatever happened to the original Hippocratic oath...? "First, do no harm?"

Dr. Jordan told me to set up my Opdivo infusions with Dr. Li, and I said that I would call him.

I called Dr. Li the very next day, and he said that he could order the treatments for me at Mayo, or I could get an oncologist in Prescott to administer them. I asked how often I would need the IV, and he said I would receive treatment every three weeks. He said he could recommend another oncologist in Prescott if I needed a name, and I told him that I already see Dr. Hastings. In a shocked tone, he said that was who he was going to suggest. He told me that Dr. Hastings was the best oncologist in Prescott. I told him that it was a small town and that I already knew that but was happy to hear it from a peer. Dr. Li told me to have Dr. Hastings call him.

I put in a call to Dr. Hastings, and we set up a Telehealth visit. While waiting for this appointment, I stepped back into research mode. I tried to find everything I could on immunotherapy as a treatment for UG. I found the book "The Breakthrough" by Charles Graeber and learned all about the history of immunotherapy. It was fascinating. Some early observers have claimed that unexplained remissions from UGs were due to an immune response by the patient from another infection. Only now can we substantiate such observations by laboratory methods and rationally use immunological procedures to prevent, diagnose, and treat UG. It is clear there is a vital role for this modality of UG treatment.

Immunotherapy appears to have a far better chance of success within the framework of whole-body therapy. Unfortunately, it has taken a back seat over the years to Chemo, Radiation, and Surgery. Immunotherapy fundamentally differs from all the other current UG treatments. It works with our body's immune system to help it to recognize UG. UG uses tricks to hide from our immune system. That is why it is so deadly. UG does not announce itself with a fever or body aches or show any symptoms. It sometimes grows for years before it is discovered. For many people, the first they heard of immunotherapy was when President Jimmy Carter had a miraculous recovery with a new drug called a checkpoint inhibitor. These new drugs blocked the checkpoints that UG uses to evade our immune systems. In 2015 at 91 years old, he was cured of aggressive UG, which had spread to his liver and brain. These new drugs have opened the door to a brand-new type of treatment that addresses the patient rather than the disease. Unfortunately, many of these drugs are stacked up and waiting for FDA approval while patients die. They do not have the time to wait. UG is complicated, and not all patients respond to the new immunotherapies, but it is a breakthrough compared to the lack of success with current conventional treatments. There are now combinations of drugs that are working in certain, more stubborn UGS. In addition to Checkpoint Inhibitors like PDL1's, there are now Adoptive Cell Therapies, Monoclonal Antibodies, Oncolytic Virus Therapies, Cancer Vaccines, and Immune System Modulators. As of 2017, the FDA had approved 32 different immunotherapies for patients with UG.

Before I talked to Dr. Hastings, I made a particularly important call. I called Dr. Julius Strauss from the National Cancer Institute at the National Institute of Health in Bethesda, MD. He answered his phone on the second ring, and I reminded him of the emails and phone calls we traded last year. I told him that I had the Nigro protocol and that I had had a hard time with chemo and never got into the Opdivo trial because of that. We discussed my metastases and my most recent scans. I told him that my doctors now wanted me to go on the Opdivo. I told him that I had been reading up on immunotherapy and that I heard that some of the combination trials were having better results than the single agents, and he said that was true. I told him that I would feel better knowing that my drugs were specifically targeted at HPV UGs. He said that my chance of Nivolumab working for me was about 30%.

I was not surprised because I had already looked up the statistics from the last Nivolumab trial, specifically on Anal Cancer patients. Dr. Strauss said that they hoped to beat those odds by about 20%. They were hoping for a 50-60% response rate. It is not a cure rate, but a response rate, as they will no longer call it a cure after metastases. I wanted in! He said the trial was perfect for me but then said I would have to have a current scan and blood tests to see if I qualified. He thought, based on my interpretation of the last scan, that I would. He said I would need one lymph node to measure at least 1.5 cm on one side. I had that. He reminded me that the drugs were experimental and that this was phase I for the combination of the three drugs and phase II for the main agent. I asked him how many patients were in the trial, and he said that I would be the seventh and that we were grouped in three phases and that if I were chosen, I would be the first patient in the second phase. I asked how the other patients were doing in the first phase and what side effects they were having, and he said they were getting rashes that were manageable with steroid creams. He said that they were also getting flu-like symptoms for a few days after treatment. He wanted me to understand other more serious side effects from the main drug, M7824, the most serious being bleeding.

"What kind of bleeding," I asked?

"It is mostly minor, like bleeding gums. One patient in phase one might need a blood transfusion. I will keep you informed on his status. We must resolve his issues to the team's satisfaction before we can enroll any phase two patients. I feel confident that we will get this resolved, but I cannot say exactly when that will be."

This patient was bleeding rectally and had the same UG that I had. He asked me if I had any rectal bleeding post-treatment, and I told him that I did due to fissures, but only occasionally. He said that I would bleed more with the M7824. The last thing he told me regarding side effects was that I could develop any type of over-active immune condition.

Dr. Strauss continued, "Because the drugs put your immune system into high gear, you can get colitis or potentially any condition ending in "itis."

"Oh really? Can you tell me how serious that can get?"

He explained that my medications could cause a cytokine reaction, and if not controlled, I might have to withdraw from the trial. He said that most conditions so far have been mild and treatable. This was all very frightening to me. But still, for me, not as frightening as more chemotherapy or radiation. I liked how honest Dr. Strauss was with me, and I decided to put my efforts into getting into this trial. Our last concern was how long I was willing to wait for treatment. My enrollment in the trial would be on hold until this patient's bleeding condition resolved to the satisfaction of the benefactors. It could be months. I decided to go back to Dr. Li and ask him his opinion on this trial and its benefits as he seemed the most suited to answer this question. I was hoping as much anyway.

I spoke to Ben briefly about my plans, and he looked surprised. Surprised that I would travel, take experimental drugs, and that I even found the trial. He said that I should do whatever I had to do. While waiting to speak with Li, I decided to reach out to Dr. Kumar. Dr. Kumar was the oncologist I saw when Dr. Kelson misdiagnosed my rash and other chemotherapy side effects. Dr. Singh gave me his personal phone number, so I texted him. He told me that the combination trial could potentially give me better odds. He recommended that I get genomic testing done first, and that test would reveal which trials/drugs may benefit me the most. Hmmm? Why hadn't Mayo suggested this? I didn't even know that this was available to me. Of course, I immediately googled 'genomic testing for cancer.' Advanced Genomic Testing is designed to help identify the DNA alterations that drive the growth of certain UGS. This information can help identify what is unique to a particular UG and target which therapies are best designed to fight it. It's the test used before Targeted Therapies are offered. This Genomic Testing is done using the biopsy sample from the tumor. Mine was at Mayo. It was now a year and a half old. Was it still good? I then emailed Dr. Strauss and asked him if it would help if I got tested. He said that he would be most interested in seeing those results.

My call with Dr. Hastings was very brief. He said that he had my recent PET scan and that he was sorry about my diagnosis. He said that he would be happy to work with Dr. Li's orders and administer the Nivolumab. I told him that I was now considering enrollment in a Clinical Trial through NIH. He was silent for a while, and I continued. "It is for another immunotherapeutic combination that is specifically designed for HPV Cancers." He seemed intrigued. I told him the drug did not have a name yet. "It is known as M7824 if you want to look it up. It is combined with IL12 and a new HPV Vaccine which I could not remember the name of. He suggested that I speak again with Dr. Li and get back to him. By this, I assumed that he thought Dr. Li's experience was superior to his on this subject. I told him that I planned to do just that.

Dr. Li called me the next morning, and we discussed the trial. I gave him the exact names of the drugs and asked him if he knew about any of them. He did not admit his lack of knowledge, but it was evident when he changed the topic and asked me if I was comfortable traveling during Covid. I said that I was planning to stay with my daughter in Chicago and travel from there because it would be a much shorter flight. I could tell he was surprised that I was considering flying back and forth every two weeks. I asked him if I would benefit from the combination trial, and he said that all checkpoint inhibitors work basically the same way. I told him that this one was a combination of a checkpoint inhibitor and a TGF Beta known only as M7824 and that I would also be getting two other agents, the NHS-IL12 and the PDS-101. He admitted that the combination therapies were doing better than the single agents as far as response rates went. I told him that I wanted to enroll in this trial, provided he did not know of any other combination trial as good or better. He said that he did not. I couldn't believe that he did not offer to check some databases for me to make sure that I was not missing something. I couldn't believe that he did not tell me about this trial already. I had to find it myself. Why was this not part of his job?

I was hoping that he would investigate the trial that I was about to sign up for to ensure it was safe, but I knew he would not. I gave him Dr. Strauss's phone number, but I knew that he would not call him. I explained how Dr. Strauss told me that my chances for a cure could be increased substantially, and he said nothing. *How do you say nothing after that?* I asked him what he thought about my waiting up to a few months before starting immunotherapy or if he thought I should go on the Nivolumab now and then enter the trial later. He said that I could wait, but if the pain in my legs and back got any worse or any other symptoms arose, I should call him. Before leaving, I asked him to order a Genomic Test on my biopsy. He reluctantly said that he would. This was not protocol. I told him that I needed my last few scans sent to NIH, and I let him know that I would need one more CT scan right before enrollment. I felt like Mayo Clinic's Medical Oncology Department had let me down once again.

I was taking control of my health and treatment in a way that I had never done before. I could not think of anyone who knew my disease better than I did myself at this time.

I phoned my children and told them about my PET scan and the metastasis and explained it all to them as best I could. I could tell that they had no idea what I was talking about. All they heard was that my UG was back. They wondered why I was still upbeat. I explained how the trial was specifically geared toward my UG and gave me a better chance for a cure. My daughter agreed that I could stay with her in her basement apartment that she was currently rehabbing. She was in a new home (which we helped her purchase) and living with her boyfriend. Her house is in a busy neighborhood on Chicago's near west side. During my recovery, she searched for a house and looked primarily at three flats or two flats with basements that could be converted to Air B and B's. While bedridden, I often scoured the real estate sites for new listings since the market in Chicago for these properties was hot. She closed on her two-flat just after the new year. Unfortunately, shortly after purchasing the property, she lost her job.

Michelle works in Experiential Marketing, and she makes her living running large events. People were no longer attending large events. The new guidelines now had us wearing masks in public and maintaining six feet of distance from each other. Although I had already seen several pictures, I was looking forward to seeing her house in person and helping her finish the lower level. I just could not give her a definite date at this time, and I had no idea how long I would need to stay with her. Having a place to stay in Chicago was a huge help to me during Covid, but I would not outstay my welcome.

"You are not alone…Guideposts are all around you. Watch, listen and sense the answers unfold."

Karen Garvey

Chapter 25

Balance

The warm weather did not kill the airborne virus as some predicted. Covid was rampant, and the death toll was mounting daily. Hospitals were experiencing shortages in personal protective equipment, and ventilators were in high demand. Some states had plenty while others could not obtain even the essentials. I couldn't believe what I heard and saw on the news each night. I knew that I couldn't chance contracting the virus, so I stayed away from people as much as possible. It was now mandatory to leave the pins in at our golf club and use our own rakes for the bunkers. We no longer shared carts with anyone other than our immediate family members, and after our rounds, we gave each other elbow bumps or tapped our putters together. We were lucky that golf was one of the few sports that we could still enjoy and maintain our distance from others in an outside environment. I stopped attending poker club and socializing with friends long before most. I now had plenty of time to research and work on my health.

My thirst for knowledge continued, and I read another book suggested by more than a few survivors on both my Square One and Anal Cancer sites. I looked for others who may have gone through a similar diagnosis when I posted that my Anal Cancer had metastasized to my lungs and para-aortic lymph nodes. Only a few ladies responded, and two of them told me that I had to read Jane McLelland's book, *How to Starve your Cancer?* They said that she had Metastatic Cervical Cancer and survived it by treating herself with diet, supplements, and some specific repurposed drugs. Because Cervical Cancer was so similar to my own UG, I was intrigued. I immediately looked it up. Unfortunately, it was not available as an Audible book, so I had to wait for Amazon to deliver. I immediately ripped the package open and started to devour the contents. I was warned that it would get extraordinarily complex toward the end, and the book did not disappoint. This book was amazing! Jane was given a terminal diagnosis with only a few weeks to live. She threw herself into research. She already had some medical knowledge as a Chartered Physiotherapist. She wasn't trying to cure her UG. Jane's approach was to stop it from growing. She dug up old and new research, and with the help of her oncologist, they worked to metabolically starve her UG from the nutrients it relied on to grow. She discovered a unique cocktail of old drugs and repurposed them to starve the UG stem cells effectively. She also used various supplements to add to her UG starvation protocol. I was already taking many of the same supplements –things like Curcumin, D3, Quercetin, IVC, Berberine, and Naltrexone. She also did Ozone treatments, just like I did. Jane took my protocol a step further.

This is an absolute oversimplification, but she discovered that she needed to stop all the possible fueling pathways for her UG. As a background, Jane had first been diagnosed with Cervical UG in 1994, and after surgery and relentless rounds of chemotherapy, it returned to her lungs five years later. She was only 35 years old when she was told she had 12 weeks to live. She was determined to find a cure.

In Chapter 22, Jane breaks it down into four simple moves. Diet, Exercise, Supplements, and Off-Label Drugs. I understood a lot about the first three, but what exactly did she mean by "Off-Label Drugs"? It was confusing but here goes.

She studied our UG and discovered it was fueled primarily by glucose, as most UGS are. All the possible pathways needed blocking, and she and her oncologist determined that diet and supplements could not achieve this independently. Her protocol included Aspirin and Dipyridamole to help stymie the abnormal cell signaling. One such abnormal cell signaling, Wnt signaling, controlled by miR-34a, is an epigenetically controlled micro-RNA strand with antiviral activity. Deregulation of Wnt signaling is responsible for the invasion and progression of herpes viruses. The HPV virus can manipulate and control this pathway and therefore evade host immune recognition. I realized through her research that I have a Wnt driven UG. I had to read this information several times to understand it, as it was complex, to say the least.

Dipyridamole is an old drug that is sometimes used to prevent blood clots after heart surgery. Antiplatelets have been found to reduce metastases. Jane said that her blood tests showed that her Interleukin 12 and Tumor Necrosis Factor Beta results were suppressed. I bet mine are too. These control our Natural Killer Cells. When the allergy response is raised, the Natural Killer Cells are suppressed. How could my immune system do its job when it is being bullied by a virus? One of Dr. Strauss's trial drugs was Interleukin 12, and I recalled him saying that it was made up of natural macrophages and dendritic cells. He said that my immune system needed them to recognize my UG. Could these drugs help me even more? I was convinced that I needed this trial and wanted to get on these off-label drugs immediately.

She goes on to discuss yet another repurposed drug, Metformin. Metformin is a diabetes drug that lowers your blood sugar by improving the way your body handles insulin. It increases glucose uptake in muscle cells and therefore decreases overall glucose, glutamine, and insulin levels. I needed that too. I have been trying to control my glucose through my diet, but this would be quicker.

Then she talks about Doxycycline. Doxy is an antibiotic used for acne, from what I recall. Study results suggest that doxycycline suppresses cancer cell proliferation and primes cells for apoptosis. I read on.

Lovastatin is another drug in her protocol. Statins block the cell's ability to make cholesterol for new cell walls. Fats are just another nutrient source for UG.

She also took an antiviral medication called Mebendazole. This drug could help block new UG blood vessel growth. I was so inspired, excited, and full of hope. I could not contain my optimism. I knew that I needed to speak with Dr. Zander. I hoped he would understand the reasoning behind Jane's protocol, and he was the only doctor that would possibly give me prescriptions for the drugs. I could not get them without a prescription, or so I thought.

During my next vitamin C infusion, I stopped by his office. I talked so quickly, and even through my mask, he could see how excited I was. He reacted very favorably to my questionable description of Jane's protocol, and he understood some of its merits. He said he would read the book immediately and get back to me.

While waiting for Dr. Zander to read the book, I revisited the difficult chapters and found that a clinic out of London had endorsed it. They were called the Care Oncology Group. When I googled them, I discovered that they had just recently opened a US chapter. Their website was full of information on the drug protocol. It was not exactly what Jane took, but it was similar. They offered a combination of four different off-label drugs, but you had to register with them as a patient, and the cost was 800 dollars. I immediately signed up to get more information. A nurse would call me to discuss my enrollment. It was handled very similarly to a trial. While I waited for the nurse to call me, Dr. Zander called back, and he was excited about the book. He thanked me for bringing it to his attention. I got chills when I knew that an MD was embracing my crazy find. I felt like we were onto something. I told him about the Care Oncology website, and he took note of that as well. He said that he would be happy to prescribe three out of four of the drugs. He was not convinced that the statin was a good idea. He said that in some cases, statins could make cancer worse. I got three scripts from him and started to take the drugs immediately. He told me that the doses were extremely low and that the drugs have been around for so long and are considered very safe for long-term use. It was funny when I took them to my pharmacy. I could only get one of the three scripts that day. I had to wait for the Dipyridamole. They said it was an incredibly old drug and that most doctors were now prescribing others. They also did not have access at all to the antiviral, Mebendazole. I spoke with others on my Facebook group, and they said that Fenbendazole was the same drug and that I could substitute.

Fenbendazole, or FenBen as it is often called, is a drug used by Veterinarians to treat intestinal parasites in pets. It is an antiviral. I immediately ordered the FenBen from Amazon, making sure to get the exact type recommended by others. I also joined a new Facebook group called the Fenbendazole group. They had over 9,000 members who believed that intestinal parasites were often the culprits for UG. If most of your immune system is in your abdomen, removing any intestinal parasites taking up residence made sense. You may find this outrageous, but I immediately started to drink the packaged powder dissolved in a glass of water each morning. My research had shown that it was perfectly harmless and could indeed benefit me, and Dr. Zander confirmed that, as it was one of the three drugs that he was on board with.

After speaking to the nurse from Care Oncology, I decided to spend the money on enrollment and make an appointment to speak with one of their oncologists. My 800 dollars covered a one-hour consultation, unlimited access to the nurses, and three short follow-ups. If that was what the doctor ordered, all four drugs would need to be ordered through them and paid for upfront. They would be mailed to me. I was told that insurance would not cover them but that the cost was minimal. Unfortunately, they wanted me to order a three-month supply at one time. My consultation with the oncologist was interesting. His name was Dr. Huang, and he had spent many years as a medical oncologist prescribing and administering chemotherapy to patients. When he was offered the position with Care Oncology, he did not hesitate to join them. He said that chemo and the drug protocol could work synergistically to increase the chances of remission or cure in many stubborn UGS. Their own five-year study had proven this. Unfortunately, it is said that chemotherapy alone works in only 6-8% of UG cases. That's dismal. This oncologist knew that his patients were dying, and he was looking for a new way to treat them. Many of COC's patients were late-stage and doing a combination of both. He did not have much experience with Anal UG, but he did with Cervical Cancer, and after reviewing my files, he recommended the standard four-drug protocol. I asked him if it could be used alongside immunotherapy, and he said "absolutely." He had a few patients doing both. I ordered the Mebendazole to replace my FenBen and the statin drug Atorvastatin through Care Oncology. This was against Dr. Zander's advice, but Dr. Huang assured me that the statin was necessary to block an important fueling pathway.

I regularly contacted Dr. Strauss, but I did not tell him about my repurposed drugs. I simply told him that I was throwing everything I could at my UG. I'm sure he assumed that I was one of those alternative quacks. I could not chance telling him about the details of my newest protocol for fear that he might reject me for his trial. Many of the members of my

Square One group treat their UGs with only herbs and tinctures. They are not fans of any pharmaceuticals. They trust that the Lord will guide them. I do not fit that description. I try to look at the overall picture. I agree that the pharmaceutical industry is corrupt in many ways, but there are good scientists and important discoveries that we cannot live without. I also know that many of those discoveries are derived from powerful herbs. It was a balancing act. I already suspected that I would have to take myself off the repurposed drugs once the trial began. I could not chance any adverse interactions. I just wanted to keep my UG weak during this waiting period. Just like the name implies, my plan was to control its growth.

Dr. Jordan called Dr. Strauss, and they discussed what scans he needed and briefly talked about the treatments I would receive. Dr. Jordan told him that he would be available if any stubborn nodes did not respond. Wow! My radiation oncologist took the time to call Dr. Strauss. This was something that Dr. Li should have done since he was my medical oncologist. I would think that he would have been more than curious about a new immunotherapy combination offering more hope to patients. Dr. Strauss kept me updated on the patient with the rectal bleeding. He did have the blood transfusion, and he was put back on the trial meds after a brief delay. It sounded more and more like the trial would be moving forward to the next phase. We discussed an August 18 start date.

I set up my CT scan at Mayo for early August. This was to be my final entrance scan. It had to be done within 30 days of my enrollment. NIH now had all my other scans and labs. Dr. Strauss reviewed them and said that I looked like the perfect candidate for the trial.

I continued my supplements, IV's, ozone, juicing diet, off-label drugs, sauna, meditation, exercise, and the occasional golf round. My days were full. I spent my evenings with Ben and the dogs. I knew that I would soon be moving to Chicago and that I might possibly be away from them for many months.

The weeks flew by, and I return to Mayo for the umpteenth time for my final CT scan. It has been agreed that my results will be forwarded to NIH, and Dr. Strauss will call me with those as soon as he reviews them. When he calls me, there is a change in his voice. He gets right to the point and tells me that my lymph nodes have shrunk. That's great news, I think to myself, but then he tells me that I don't have "measurable" UG. Some of the nodes are back to normal, and some are just shy of the minimum requirement of 1.5cm. He still feels sure that it is UG as there are also the same spots in my chest and lungs, and a couple of those have now merged. They are still not considered measurable enough for trial entry.

I hang up and immediately call Dr. Jordan and ask him if he still thinks I should get the Nivolumab or if I should wait and rescan, and he says, "definitely." I still need to do something. My nodes are smaller, but only slightly. I wonder if my protocols are controlling my UG. It's been three months, and with metastatic UG, they should have grown.

Now I don't know what to do. Do I continue with my off-label drugs and supplements? How long can I keep it up? Should I cut it to just the repurposed drugs? At least those are cheap. It's costly for me to do it all. I think about others that don't have the opportunities that I have and I wish the system worked differently. Why won't insurance or medicare pay for alternative therapies instead of the ridiculously expensive chemotherapy, radiation, and surgeries? It would make so much more sense to pay for preventative measures, but that is not our reality. If I'm going to do immunotherapy, I want the ones in the trial. I decided to email Dr. Strauss again:

Dear Dr. Strauss,

My phone just reminded me that I was due to start the trial today. I was all set to drive to Chicago last week and fly to Bethesda for treatment today. I was wondering if you could maybe take one more look at my previous scan from Mayo and compare it to the August scan. To me, it looks like there is more activity in my chest and lungs now, and the nodes are only slightly smaller. They measured 1.5cm in May, so why would they get smaller? Could they be sitting at a different angle?

Dr. Jordan still wants me to go on the Opdivo, and your words keep sticking in my mind about how the M7824 could offer me better odds for a cure.

It would mean so much to me if you took just one more look. I promise not to get my hopes up.

Best Regards,
Bonnie L

Within minutes of my pressing 'send,' he called me and said he would speak with his radiologist again. He would then discuss it with the team. He reiterated that I should not count on anything.

After two days, he called again and said that I was approved for the trial. I would have to sign a lot of paperwork regarding side effects and required scanning, but I could do this when I got to NIH. I would need blood tests every two weeks, and I would need to scan every six weeks. I thought this was excessive, but I was thrilled to get into the trial. He said I could start September 1st and that my charge nurse would send me details and their travel department would set up my flights. Everything had to fall into place at the same time. The patient with the bleeding had to get things resolved, I had to get approved, and my start date had to be before September 1.

It was then a mad rush to get me to Chicago in time. I was due for my first treatment in less than ten days!

We had first entertained the thought of all of us going to Chicago, but quickly tossed that idea aside. Michelle's garden apartment is much too small to accommodate all of us. Then I considered taking Pita with me, and all I could think about was how sad DeeDee would be without him. I was going alone. I thought about flying there and then pictured myself without a car. Michelle assured me that I could use her car whenever I needed it. They also Uber a lot in the city. I'm old school and I wanted my car. I decided to drive. It will be a 3-day trip to get there because I won't drive more than seven or eight hours per day. I can no longer drive at night. My vision deteriorated after the chemotherapy. It is a well-known side effect that gets little attention. Ben offered to go with me and then come back, but I did not want him flying during Covid. I'm going alone. My friends think I'm nuts, but it doesn't bother me at all. I look forward to the solitude. It will give me time to think.

The word gets out that I am leaving town for a clinical trial that can last for up to a year. I get cards and phone calls wishing me a speedy recovery. My last thoughts are about Ben and how he will manage without me. I make him promise to walk the dogs twice a day. I go over the bills with him and tell him where I keep everything. Friends assure me that they will look in on him.

"Learn from yesterday, live for today, hope for tomorrow. The important thing is not to stop questioning."

Albert Einstein

Chapter 26

Tenacity

I am now on the road. It is surreal as I drive the Interstate. I stop for gas, pee, call Ben, stretch, and grab a healthy snack (which is hard to find in a gas station) when I reach 1/4 tank. I listen to Sirius radio and get emotional with any song that strikes a resemblance to my life. I start to listen to my audible books after the songs get repetitious. The last couple of hours of my daily drives are the worst. I struggle to keep alert by ramping up the volume on my radio or by sucking on sunflower seeds. I become a pro at opening them and separating the seeds from the shells. I fill my cup holder with the wet, splintered shells. My tongue gets raw from the salt, and I move on to other "keep awake" strategies, my last being ice on my eyelids. Finally, I start to see mileage signs for my exit. The hotels I picked were nowhere near as nice as the reviews and photos indicated, and they have barely any other guests. I wear a mask everywhere. I make trips back and forth from the car to gather my change of clothes and snacks for the room. If there is a local Starbucks, I stop for a Medicine Ball (a Teavana tea mixture of Jade Citrus Mint and Peach Tranquility teas with steamed fresh lemonade and honey).

I raise my voice to the large backlit menu, "A vente medicine ball with half the honey, please."

If there is a grocery store, I stop for a healthy microwavable dinner. Is that an oxymoron? I strip the bed and use my own sheets, pillow, and comforter. I want to take a bath, but I don't dare. Instead, I take a long hot shower and watch a little TV. I call Ben and Michelle, set my alarm, and head off to slumberland.

When I finally get to Chicago, I hit traffic, but it's not horrendous. I planned not to arrive during any part of Chicago's lengthy rush hour, but I forgot it's Friday night, and I hit weekend travelers and construction. There is a saying about Chicago traffic ... 'It's either winter or construction.'

Finally, I get to her house and get the tour. It is a small two-story frame with faded yellow siding and a brown asphalt roof over a hundred years old. Nothing special, but I see every bit of its potential. I couldn't see the upper apartment because she has a tenant. Her apartment is smaller than it appeared in the photos, but bright and well-kept, and I can see why she liked it. It was in move-in condition. We then make our way down to the garden apartment. I have already been warned about the low ceilings, but they are fine for me. Mark has to duck in two spots, but you can see that he is used to it. It has been freshly painted, and there is a brand-new luxury vinyl plank floor that they installed themselves. It's beautiful, but the baseboards and trim have not been reinstalled yet. The kitchen cabinets have been recently painted a gorgeous green with brushed gold hardware. It is a very trendy choice, and I admire her style. There is no countertop yet, so she placed plywood on top for my stay. Mark tells me that she cleaned for hours, especially in the bathroom. The bedroom looks comfy, but the bathroom is tiny. I wonder how I will manage with all my things. I will surely miss my bathtub as there is only one tight shower. I unpack my bags, we order dinner to be delivered by Uber Eats, and we catch up on things at her new dining room table. I have two days to settle in, and then I'm off to NIH.

The summers are beautiful in Chicago. I spend hours outside, either on the front porch or in the garden. I finally get to taste a homegrown tomato from her vines. It is just as I remembered.

"You can't get or grow tomatoes like this in Arizona," I lament.

The trees and grass are a brilliant green. It is a much more humid climate, but I like humidity. Most people complain about it, but it makes my skin feel great.

Monday comes around in no time at all. Michelle drops me off at the blue line where I will take the train to O'hare Airport. It is the fastest way to get there. After a long and exhaustive day of travel in the middle of Covid, I arrive in DC at the Ronald Reagan Washington National Airport, where I am supposed to meet an NIH-hired cab. After a few minutes, my cabbie shows up and takes me to my hotel. It is late afternoon, and the ride to Bethesda takes me down Washington Memorial Parkway through dense green forest preserves that occasionally allow me glimpses of the Potomac River. I have chosen the American Inn, which is conveniently close to NIH.

I make myself a hot tea, put on the news, and lie down. I am exhausted and fall asleep immediately. I wake up at about 11 pm, and I am starving, but nothing is open at that hour except a local pizza restaurant. I order the pizza online, and it is delivered downstairs. Only guests are allowed in the elevators during Covid, so I must go down to the lobby and pick it up. *What the hell?* I haven't eaten a pizza in a long time, and it is a bit cold but delicious. I eat the whole small pizza and watch a little more TV.

I clean the tub even though it looks clean. After a soothing hot bath, I get into my jammies, set my alarm, and settle down again. I wake up again at 4 am with an awful stomach ache. I shuffle through my bag for a chewable licorice tablet which acts similarly to tums. I drink a full bottle of water and cannot fall back asleep. I hope I can go number two before I have to leave. My first appointment is at 8 am, so I am getting picked up at seven by the NIH shuttle. It has a regular route and stops at several hotels. After two cups of hot decaf coffee, I finally go to the bathroom. Whew! That's one thing I will not have to worry about.

The driver takes me to the wrong entrance of NIH. I can't believe how big the complex is. I can see several buildings within the interior, and the exterior is completely fenced with barbed wire and has several security entrances. The attendant tells us that we need to go to the east side. My driver takes me there, and they explain that I will need to go through security. I have my small rolling suitcase containing my laptop, sweater, water bottle, and snacks. I must walk through a metal detector, and my bag has to go through a scanner. The main hospital building is off in the distance, about two football fields away. If I want the Uber driver to take me to the door, he must go through security and have his car checked. That's ridiculous, so I instruct him just to leave me at the gate. After getting my day pass, I have to walk to the hospital, a completely uphill journey.

After going through several Covid protocols at the front entrance, I find the main lab. I am called in for my blood draw. The phlebotomist takes several brightly colored vials from the shelf and even more from inside the drawers. There is a total of 17. *Holy cow!* I have never had this many vials of blood drawn from me. She tells me it will go quickly, and if I feel lightheaded afterward, to let her know. She explains that the "research draw" is only once per month. So, every other visit will be 17 vials, and the rest of the time, it will be 5. I wonder how many scientists will look at my blood and how long they keep it.

I find the right elevators and head up to the 12th floor, where several patients are waiting. I look around and notice that many are not speaking English. These patients are from all over the world. There is a child in a wheelchair slumped over, a young pregnant woman, and a myriad of others. There is a cooler at the front with a sign that says, "help yourself." It is filled with juice and water bottles. On a table next to it are several brown paper bags marked either breakfast or lunch. I take one marked breakfast and shuffle through it to find yogurt, a muffin, spoon, and napkin. I sign in, and they give me paperwork to fill out. After returning the paperwork, they provide me with an armband and ask me to take a seat. I pick on my muffin, and finally I am called.

My first stop is with an intake nurse who weighs me and takes my vitals. I then go back to the waiting room and wait for my name to be called again. The clinic rooms are old and filled with furniture and equipment that looks like it is from the '50s. For some reason, it reminds me of *One Flew Over the Cuckoo's Nest,* and I imagine my nurse will look like Nurse Ratchet. Finally, she arrives, and she is welcoming and chatty. I like her immediately—no resemblance to Nurse Ratchet. We go over some paperwork, and then I am seen by a fellow who gives me a quick exam and asks me several questions.

Then a man comes in, and my nurse stands up to greet him. I am introduced to Dr. Sater. Dr. Strauss is not in today. Dr. Sater is one of my main team of physicians. He hands me his business card, which tells me he is an oncologist and immunologist with a Ph.D. He seems to be in a hurry, and we have a lot of paperwork to go over. He spends most of his time talking about potential side effects. We go through my list of current medications, and he sees that they are all supplements. I have just stopped my COC protocol, so I do not even bother to bring those up. Even though I already know from earlier conversations with Dr. Strauss, I ask Dr. Sater if I can continue with my supplements. He is even more strict than Dr. Strauss and explains that I must be only on the trial drugs and those explicitly approved for any side effects. Otherwise, he explains, we will not know exactly what is causing any particular side effect. He explains that I will be getting all three biologics today, and for my next visit, it will be the M7824 alone. The M7824 will be given by IV. I ask if they can use my port, and he says they can, but only if it is made from titanium. We determine that mine is not. I have this port that I got for my Vitamin C treatments, and I cannot even use it for immunotherapy. They apologize for this inconvenience. The other two drugs are administered by injection. The PDS101 HPV vaccine will be given in two separate syringes, and the Interleukin 12 vaccine will be just one shot. They will give them to me in a large muscle like my thigh. If I decide to do the trial, I will come back tomorrow for treatment. I was already aware of this and knew that this would be a two-day trip due to the paperwork and enrollment procedures. He goes over the side effects once again and asks me if I want to make any other phone calls before making this decision. Hmmm? I guess not, I think to myself. I sign the forms, and Dr. Sater signs off on them as well.

Back at the hotel, I plan my early dinner. A lot of restaurants are closed due to Covid. Instead, I pick up a salad and baked sweet potato at a trendy cafe within walking distance. Downtown Bethesda is lovely with many small shops, and I wish I was here for a vacation and not for treatment in a clinical trial, but it is what it is. I stop at Starbucks on my way back.

The next morning, I wake up early, mask up and catch the shuttle outside on time. I have checked out and have my full carry-on bag with me this time. I will go straight to the airport after my treatments. There are two other patients at my hotel who are waiting for the NIH shuttle as well. I figure this hotel does most of its business from NIH patients. There are a lot more occupants this time. The morning shuttle is busiest. We all go through security and then reboard the shuttle. This time I get dropped off at the door. My first stop is at the clinic to meet with Dr. Sater again. He reviews my blood tests with me and signs off on treatment. Any time I get treatment, I will go through this same procedure. I am told to check-in at the Day Hospital on the west side of floor 3. I find out that there are several day hospitals after first checking in at the wrong one. I check-in, and they take my cell phone number. They ask me to stay on the premises and tell me that the wait can be up to three hours. That seems excessive, but I wait. I read, eat snacks, and walk around the hospital with my carry-on in tow. This time, I take in the photos on the walls and admire the beautiful quilts displayed in cases throughout my floor. There are several comfortable waiting areas, and I check out all of them before finding my favorite. When I am called in, I get a personal nurse who escorts me to a reclining chair. There are several rooms, and each room has four recliners. They look like hospital rooms with all the equipment but with recliners instead of beds.

The nurse is a sweet older woman who makes sure that I am comfortable and have something to eat. She informs me that the HPV vaccine will be given in two separate shots. She then checks the side of the syringes against her paperwork and calls in another nurse to repeat those same procedures. They ask my name and date of birth each time and check my wristband. She jabs the first needle in unexpectedly, and I yelp from the pain. It is a huge needle. She apologizes and asks if I would rather know it's coming. I tell her to choose. Then it happens again in a different spot about two inches from the other. She first measured to make sure it was far enough away from the other. It hurts like hell. Then she goes to the other leg and gives me the IL12 shot. It is a much smaller needle, and I feel little pain from it. She tells me to leave my pants down for a few minutes to ensure there is no reaction. I immediately start to develop two very red lumps, which she tells me is normal. After a time, she lets me get dressed and pulls back the curtain. The infusion of M7824 takes two hours. I am finally done and have been warned that I may get flu-like symptoms that could start in the next 12 -24 hours. I now have to rush because my flight is leaving out of Reagan National at 7 pm. I call Michelle and Ben and give them the rundown. Michelle says she will pick me up at O'hare.

I get into Chicago at 9 pm. I'm still feeling fine, but my leg hurts and is now swollen and black and blue at the vaccine injection sites. We order food for dinner, and I tell them all about my trip. Michelle says she wants to go with me next time and drive there and see some sites. I have never been to DC and look forward to that. She also has a friend who lives there who may have an empty apartment we can stay in. She is thinking of it as a vacation, but for me, it is not that. I have to wait to find out how I will feel with these new drugs.

I retire to my garden apartment. After a few hours in bed, I start to get cold. Her thermostat controls my apartment. We share the same air conditioning, so I cannot shut it off. It is too late to call her, so I pile on more blankets and start up a small space heater that I brought with me from home. The space heater helps a little, but I am still cold. I start to get achy joints, and now my stomach hurts. I am nauseous, but it is not as bad as with chemo. I finally fall back asleep. When I wake up, I am sweating profusely, but it is a cold sweat. I am also shaking like a leaf. I reluctantly call Michelle and wake her up. I tell her that I cannot get warm. While I take a hot shower, she closes the vents and covers them with magnetized pads to prevent the air from escaping. I feel no better at all.

Nothing can warm me. I show her my hands and how awful they are shaking. I cannot stop the shaking. She brings me a second space heater and shuts off the air conditioning to the house. I apologize for being an inconvenience. I pile on more clothes and blankets and finally fall back asleep. I wake up again after a few hours, and my clothes are completely soaked. I am freezing, so I change and crawl back into the covers. I fall asleep again, only to wake yet again after a couple of hours completely drenched. I take another hot shower and change clothes and sheets. This happens four times! I email Dr. Strauss, and he calls me back within minutes. I explain my side effects, and he is concerned but tells me that this is from the IL12. He says that my next visit will be better because it will be only the M7824. He says my symptoms should subside in another day at the most and that I should drink a lot of water and take the recommended Tylenol every four hours. I take the Tylenol immediately, and within a couple of hours, the chills are gone. I am still achy, but this I can handle. The Tylenol helps a lot, so I take them every four hours. I have never had chills like this before. There was nothing I could do to warm up. I shook uncontrollably. Even in a hot shower, I was cold. Michelle brought me a small stool to sit on in the shower, and I sat there with the hot water running on my back. I was afraid I was using up all their hot water, but it felt so good.

I finally came out of my funk. I spent the next day shopping for groceries, helping Michelle around the house, and catching up with old friends. I have plenty of friends in Chicago that I haven't seen for a long time. We took walks in the forest preserve, and I even golfed one day with some girls I haven't seen in years. They set me up with some borrowed clubs, and I played a course where I used to play in a league. We have dinner later at a sports bar with a large outdoor seating area. The fall weather was unusually warm, and people in Chicago take advantage of these days knowing full well they are numbered. Life in the big city is different. The virus was hurting so many small businesses. I hoped they could recover someday because that was what made Chicago special. It was all the small independent stores, bars, and restaurants that made it so vibrant. There were no street festivals or events. We did our best to socialize with small outdoor groups, in our masks, of course.

Two weeks passed quickly, and we decided to pass on the road trip and plan it for early October on a treatment week that did not include the IL12!

On my next trip to DC, my friend dropped me off at the airport on a Monday, and Michelle planned to pick me up on Tuesday night. I tried a different hotel this time. This one had a Starbucks in the lobby. It was a Hyatt, and I got a room with a huge king-sized bed. I walked to Whole Foods and splurged on some great healthy snacks for dinner. I jacked the heat up to 76, took a luxurious bath, and laid down to watch a movie. I fell asleep and forgot to set my alarm. I woke up and scrambled to get ready and packed up. I was late for the shuttle, so I had to call an Uber again.

I rushed up the steps with all my gear and got to the lab about 15 minutes late. It was not a problem. After my blood draws, I headed up to the clinic, hoping to meet Dr. Strauss this time. He was not available, and I had another doctor from my team. This time it was Dr. Floudas. He was very personable. We talked about the weather, golf, and Covid and discussed my side effects from my last treatment. He said that I would not experience those extreme chills this time. He approved my treatment for today, and I headed off to the Day Hospital for what I thought would be easy since it was just the one drug this time. After waiting for three hours, they called me in, and this time, I had a nurse I did not like. He seemed like he thought he was too good for his job. If I had to guess, I would say that he was working his way up to another career. After hooking me up to the IV, he left the room, and I started to feel a tightness in my chest. I didn't want to use the call button yet, so I waited to see if it would get better or go away. Within another minute or two, I started getting severe chest pains and had a hard time breathing. I pushed my call button, and it took a few minutes longer for my nurse to arrive. I must have had a panicked look on my face because he immediately dialed back the IV to shut the medicine flow. My symptoms subsided very quickly to a more manageable level. I explained my symptoms to him, and he said I should have shut my IV off at the source. Well, maybe he should have told me that before he left the room.

Dr. Floudas must have gotten a call while seeing patients and rushed up to see me because he arrived within 15 minutes. He said that I must have had an allergic reaction to the drug. I asked why it didn't happen two weeks ago, and he said that my body accepted it the first time because it didn't know what was coming, but now it was saying, "hell no, I know what you are trying to give me, and I don't want any part of it." He was amusing me with his explanation, but I was terrified to take that drug again. He said that we would have to increase my Benadryl. They gave me an additional dose of 50mg through my IV, and I immediately felt a rush of what I thought would be nausea but immediately turned to a sense of calm, and then I got quite woozy. The nurse then started up the M7824, and my body tolerated it. I felt the chest tightness but to a much lesser degree. It was tolerable. It was ordered that I be given the drug over three hours instead of two. I wondered if I would make my flight. I kept busy during the three hours. I ordered food and got caught up on my phone calls, texts, and emails. While I was there, I overheard in the chair next to me that they were administering an HPV Vaccine. After they pulled the curtain back, I saw that it was a woman about my age and build, and we started talking. We were the exact same age. Her birthday was one day before mine. Our husbands both had prostate cancer, and we each had two grown children. Lastly, we shared the same diagnosis. The only difference being that she had surgery to remove her tumor, and I had the Nigro protocol. Her metastases were in her liver. She had started on my trial and then had to be taken off the M7824 because she got a rash that turned into skin cancer. *Wow!* Now she was getting just the vaccine. We could have talked all day, but she had to leave, my bag was almost empty, and I would be rushing to catch a plane. I had a cab set up to rush me to the airport, and I barely made it.

About a day or two after my return to Chi-town, I started to notice my skin was very itchy. At night when I didn't realize what I was doing, I scratched my skin raw in a couple of places. It got to where it was extremely itchy all day and night. My neck started getting a thick rash all over it, and there were patches here and there on my body. Nothing helped. I called Dr. Strauss and he answered straight away. He told me to start taking Benadryl every four hours. He also prescribed me a steroid cream for the worst areas. He told me to use that cream very sparingly. I did, and it helped a little. The itch never went away completely, but it became more tolerable. I told him that I met Jeannie, and he said that her case was unusual and that most patients just had the itchy rash, and the creams and Benadryl took care of it. I hoped that would be the case for me, and I hoped also that Jeannie could get back into the trial. It sounded like that was her goal if she could only find the right medication to control her skin issues.

Another thing I noticed after my second treatment was that my back and legs were no longer painful. I wondered if the drugs might be working, and then I thought no way it could happen this fast and then just chalked it up to my not playing as much golf.

The next visit came quickly, and I felt like an experienced frequent flyer. I ordered the cabs to pick me up and chose the hotel that I liked best. We controlled my allergic reaction to the M7824 by high dose IV Benadryl and infusing it over three hours. I developed another set of rashes and flulike symptoms from the trio of drugs. I now knew I could control those with medication. I went out and purchased giant bottles of Extra Strength Tylenol and Benadryl. I took two Tylenol every four hours for the first few days, and it kept the flu-like symptoms and chills at bay. I controlled the continuing rashes as needed with the Benadryl and steroid creams. I had a bad stomach ache the next day and phoned Dr. Strauss again. I pleaded with him to let me take my pre and probiotics. I reminded him of our conversation before my entrance into the trial and how he said he would consider allowing certain supplements only after he got a handle on my side effects. I brought up the book I had read by Dr. Williams and how he insisted that pre and probiotic supplements were pivotal to his patient's success with immunotherapy, especially those that held Inulin and Bifidobacterium. He caved and said I could go back on them. *Yay!*

Michelle and I left early on a Monday morning for my third treatment. We were driving, and it was going to take us 10.5 hours. We each took a stint and stopped for gas and snacks along the way. We checked into a hip boutique hotel in downtown DC and ate dinner in their restaurant with an outside eating area. The weather was outstanding. The food and atmosphere were both great. She dropped me off at NIH the next morning, and I spent the entire day there while she rode bikes with her friend. After my infusion, she picked me up and we stopped at the Lincoln Memorial on the way back. We didn't have time to do much else before dark. I called Ben, and he said that he went there as a kid and remembered touching Lincoln's shoe. I told him that now you can't even get close to his shoe as it is barricaded off all around the statue.

From the top of the steps, we could see down to the Reflecting Pool and National Mall. Of course, we saw the White

House and went to the Smithsonian and had dinner at her friend's house. It was a great trip, and I felt surprisingly good except for the itchy skin. Then on the last day, I got some bloody diarrhea, which of course, freaked me out. I called Dr. Strauss. He said that he figured it would happen and that I just needed to keep an eye on it. It could bleed, but it should not pour out of me, was how he put it. I didn't really understand exactly how much blood was acceptable. To me, any seemed like too much. He then explained that more than three tablespoons were the cutoff for a day, and more than what I would have had with menstruation in a week was too much. That made a little more sense.

On my fourth visit to NIH, my labs were bad. I finally got to meet the man himself—the lead investigator. Dr. Strauss was a much younger man than I pictured in my mind. He had a manicured beard and a nervous laugh that sometimes came out at inappropriate times. I liked him and enjoyed joking with him so I could hear his laugh. I was shocked when he told me that they would have to withhold treatment this time because my liver enzymes were high. He told me that the M7824 could sometimes cause this and that they would go down before my next visit. I was disappointed and asked why it had not happened the first few times. He didn't know the answer. We talked about my other side effects like the bleeding and rashes, and then he told me that the team was lowering the dose on the IL12 by half. Not just for me but for all the patients from now on. We were the guinea pigs on dosing. I was concerned that I would have to skip all of my meds, but he said he would still send me for the vaccine and IL12. I told him about my back and leg pain being gone and asked if treatments might be helping me already. Not wanting to get me too optimistic, he simply said, "Let's wait and see." My scan was coming up on my next visit, and we would reevaluate. He casually mentioned the dosing on my Tylenol for the flu-like symptoms and said that I could lower them to half of what I was taking now that the IL12 was dosed down.

I told him how much I had been taking, and he said, "Oh no, you took how much?"

I said, "I was taking 4000mg per day."

"Oh, my god," he said. "That's way too much! That's why your liver enzymes are high. Please don't take that much ever again."

I didn't think I could overdose on Tylenol, but I guess it can do damage to your liver. Unfortunately, it looks like my liver can only handle so much.

The last thing I talked to Dr. Strauss about was the vaccine. NIH had been running the Moderna trials since March, and they were due to come out soon, hopefully before the end of the year.

"What do you think about my getting the vaccine? Do you recommend it," I asked?

"Absolutely," said Dr. Strauss.

"Would I be one of the first to get the vaccine?" I asked.

"Probably not," said Dr. Strauss. "They will need to vaccinate the most at-risk first, and that will be the front-line workers, the elderly, and other essential workers."

"There are a lot of people saying that the trials have been rushed. What do you say about that?"

Dr. Strauss adjusted his mask. "The number of participants in these trials is unprecedented, and that makes them very sound. Most trials have just a few hundred participants. These trials have attracted tens of thousands."

"You should just wait your turn. If you were to get the virus, you would fare better than most because of the antivirals that we have you on. But you should still get the vaccine. There are very few people that we will recommend against getting it."

"I thought maybe you could put in a good word for me with Fauci," I said jokingly.

I then sent him the 'Fauci on The Couchi' meme that was going around to his phone. He saw it, and I got to hear his funny laugh.

I got the treatment shots, and this time my flu-like side effects were very minimal. I still had the continued bleeding, and it bothered me a lot to have giant blood clots coming out with my stools. It was just something I had to deal with. I also had itchiness even though I did not have the M7824. Dr. Strauss told me that the drug keeps working in my body for many months, so not to worry about missing a dose. He told me that he was not concerned about my bleeding but that we would keep an eye on my labs and that I should let him know if the bleeding changed dramatically in volume.

I passed the time at Michelle's helping her with the basement apartment. We ordered and had installed white quartz countertops—what a change. The sink came with it, and she installed a beautiful, polished brass faucet all by herself after simply watching a YouTube video. I must say I was quite impressed. We painted baseboards in the garage and started to install them. This was a long and complicated process to learn how to use a miter saw. It was a lot of running back and forth from the garage where the miter saw was set up. She is a bit of a perfectionist. I know she does not get that from me. I'm all about getting things done quickly.

My fourth visit included a CT scan to evaluate my progress. It's hard for me to believe that it's been six weeks already. When I went to the clinic for my exam and scan results, I had the fellow come in first as usual, but then, instead of one doctor, I had a whole team with me. Dr. Strauss and Dr. Floudas were on a video call. Dr. Sater and Liz were there in person. I panicked and figured it was bad news. Why would all these people be here? Liz saw my panic and told me not to worry.

"This is our normal protocol for scan results," Liz explained.

"Oh, okay," I said. "I was worried that something was wrong."

"On the contrary," Dr. Strauss says, "your labs are great. Your liver enzymes are back to normal."

"That's great, and what about the scan?" I asked.

He said that he was "cautiously optimistic." He explained that the para-aortic nodes were the same, the spots in my lungs and chest are gone, and there are a couple of new lymph nodes enlarged in my chest.

I panicked.

All I could hear was that a couple of new lymph nodes were enlarged in my chest. Dr. Strauss tells me that it's good news, but I don't see it that way. I argue with him that "new nodes are bad news, right?"

He tells me that this can sometimes happen with immunotherapy. Lymph nodes can grow with inflammation while the immune system is working to kill the UG. I try to understand and share in his obvious excitement. Then I wondered if my scan at Mayo a few months ago showed enlarged nodes because of my natural immunotherapy treatments. I ask him if the other spots are really gone, and he says they are. He tells me that we will know more after the next scan, and he approves me for treatment.

Everyone asks about my scan, and I try explaining the results, but no one gets it, least of all me. If the doctors think it is a good scan, I will go along with that.

I am missing Ben, Deedee, and Pita something fierce. Ben jokingly tells me that I miss the dogs more than him. It's getting colder in Chicago, and we have had some really bad rain. I'm starting to feel claustrophobic in my little nest. Michelle and Mark are planning a trip to the east coast, and I look forward to having the whole apartment to myself. She tells me I can sleep upstairs, but I am happy just to have a bathtub, dining room, and most of all, control of the thermostat. I am now in charge of 'Lil Orange,' their cat. She is a bit skittish, but I plan to win her over when they are gone. Most animals love me.

They are taking my Audi on their trip, and I will miss it. Unfortunately, I am stuck with the Prius for the next week, where fumes from the rusted-out muffler often find their way into the car's interior. I guess I will drive with the heat on and the windows open.

I spend much of my time watching Netflix and Amazon Prime since they have no regular TVs. When I start watching bad holiday movies, I know I must find a new activity. I reach out to other survivors in my Anal Cancer Group and find out there is a subgroup for survivors that have been through clinical trials. We are a surprisingly small group. Jeannie is part of this group and a man named Tom in Canada. Tom has been through the M7824 trial, and his anal UG metastasis responded and cleared, but then it came back. I understand from Jeannie that this happened three times for him. I posted my progress online and felt relief knowing that this drug was working for someone else with my UG. When I go back to the main site, I notice this interesting exchange of texts between group members:

I just love you people sooo much. All the positive thoughts and prayers…but can we please stop sugar coating this for the newcomers. It's brutal. Period. And it's like that for an awfully long time. The side effects from chemo and radiation are awful. Can we just please tell the truth, all the doctors tell you a bit… but not the whole truth. Isn't that why we're here?

Everyone has a different pain tolerance. Treatment for me was a colostomy then six weeks of radiation with chemo every other week. Yes, it was rough, but manageable with pain meds.

I wanted to hear all the bad stuff so I knew what I might be facing.

The burns scared the hell out of me.

My radiation oncologist said that I would forget eventually. Thank goodness I have. It was horrible and I will not go through it again. I have made that clear to my caregivers. I will opt for palliative. These are my own feeling, and I don't encourage anyone else to feel this way. We all must decide for ourselves how far we want to go.

I did it all alone. It was horrible.

God Bless you all!

How people react to the initial chem-rad varies between people … some get through it while others almost drown or die. Some live fabulous lives after treatment and others suffer with poor quality lives. So many factors come into play such as staging, pre-existing conditions, etc. … so, we don't sugar coat it. but we don't say life is over as you know it either.

I'm torn on this subject, I was so scared at the start, I'm not sure I wanted the truth. Sad to say but true.

Never try to sugar coat. My oncologist said the treatment was brutal and he did not lie. I would rather be prepared for the worst and then maybe be pleasantly surprised.

I hoped with all my heart that through this trial, I could offer some alternatives to the standard surgery, chemotherapy, and radiation being recommended today. It was a brutal treatment and left horrific side effects for many patients.

A lot was happening in the news. The vaccines would receive FDA approval any day now for the Covid 19 virus, and the 2020 presidential election was about to take place. The nation was totally divided. I had Ben send me my ballot with a return receipt, and I signed and overnighted it back. Arizona was going to be a key swing state. It was what we called a 'purple state.' Michelle, Mark, and I sat glued to the TV on election night until I finally gave in and went to bed. In the morning, I woke up to the news. Trump was out. A one-term president with two impeachments on his record. Biden was going to be our new president. I hoped that he could get this virus under control and bring some unity back to our country.

My November tenth treatment went as scheduled, but after my next treatment right before Thanksgiving, I experienced my worst side effect yet. I made a big pot of chili, and it was great, but after eating a bowl of it, my mouth started to feel very strange. I thought at first that I was having an allergic reaction to the hot peppers. My lip was hot from the spices and started to feel like it was swelling up. I looked in the mirror, and now it was affecting my eye as well. Within minutes the entire left side of my face felt numb and like nothing I've ever felt before. I looked at myself in the mirror again, and it looked like I might be having a stroke.

I considered calling 911 and then decided to text Dr. Strauss. I texted him my symptoms, and he immediately called me back. He asked me to get someone to help me as soon as possible, so I called Michelle. She came down, and Dr. Strauss called back on FaceTime. He had Michelle put me through a series of tests. He asked me to raise both eyebrows as high as I could. She held the camera so that he could see my face. He asked me to smile a big smile. He asked me to shut both eyes as tight as possible and have Michelle try to open them with her fingers. My left eye was very weak and would not even close all the way. According to Michelle, my smile was very crooked, and I could not lift my eyebrow at all. Dr. Strauss said that he was 90 percent sure I had something called "Bell's Palsy." Bell's Palsy does not involve brain function. It is an impairment of the facial nerve, and it is almost always temporary. He was testing me to make sure it was that and not a stroke. They could look similar. A stroke will affect more than just your face, and it would not affect the upper face. This affected my eyebrows. He said that I could go to the clinic if I was still concerned but that he had two other patients that had gotten Bell's Palsy from the M7824. After he told me that, I felt sure of his diagnosis.

Then he went on to explain it further. He said it would go away on its own but could last for a few days or up to a few months in some cases. He said I should buy a patch for the affected eye because it would dry out from not closing it. He suggested eating on my right side and said that I would drop food and drinks from the other side of my mouth. It would be better to use a straw for drinking. I was supposed to let him know if it got much worse in the next couple of days and he could prescribe me steroids to help it go away faster. I asked him why I had to wait on the steroids, and he said that they would counteract the effects of the immunotherapy. He also said that we would have to discontinue treatment until it was fully resolved. In one patient, it had returned after treatment was reinitiated too soon.

I was not happy about stopping treatments ... again, and Dr. Strauss assured me that I would continue to benefit from the treatments I already had. Based on my last scan, he reiterated that he thought the treatments were already doing what they were supposed to do.

He said that I could come back to NIH for the HPV vaccine and the IL12 shot but that I could also just skip the next treatment altogether. We decided that with the pandemic raging, it was wise for me to cancel my next visit entirely.

After hanging up with Dr. Strauss, I googled more information on Bell's Palsy and found out that a virus can sometimes cause it, and in some cases, it has been linked to a herpes outbreak. Well, it just so happens that I had a full-blown outbreak on my bottom just that week. I started to feel it coming on a few days ago, and I felt like I was getting sick with a cold. I had the sniffles and the chills. My immune system was busy fighting my UG and my herpes/HPV, and this Bell's Palsy had some connection. I was sure of it. I texted Dr. Strauss about my speculation, but he said he didn't know about that. I sent him the article. I wished that I had not stopped taking my AHCC shiitake mushroom complex.

Ben was planning a visit for early December, and we picked dates to avoid my next treatment and symptoms. I booked his flight for December 11. This would be three days after I returned from NIH.

My Bell's Palsy got worse instead of better, and Dr. Strauss put me on a 5-day course of steroids. He said that this should speed up my recovery. He told me that they would have to cancel yet another treatment due to my Bells. I was very distraught over this, especially since I had already missed two other doses of the M7824. Once due to my elevated liver enzymes and another from the Bells. Now, this would make three. He assured me not to worry about this AT ALL. He said that the treatment works for a long time in my system. If that's true, then why do they give it every two weeks? Why not once a month? He told me that in the future, they might give it less often. That, he said, is one of many things that gets decided in a phase one trial.

The walls in my garden apartment are very thin, and on more than one occasion, I heard Michelle and Mark fighting. I heard bits and pieces of their fights and wondered if I had anything to do with those arguments. I imagined that it was not easy having your mom or your girlfriend's mom around every day for months. I tried my best to stay in my apartment as much as possible. I did not want to be a burden to them. But I was bored, and it was Covid, and while my apartment was fine for short stints, it was a bit claustrophobic. I wanted to control my own heat and air and cook meals without setting off the smoke alarm every time. I wanted to take baths, and I missed Ben and the dogs. I had secretly been contemplating going back to Arizona for a few weeks now. I did not tell Ben or Michelle, but I did mention it to Dr. Strauss. I told him that I was not going to stay in Chicago for the winter months. He assured me that I was not the only patient traveling from the west coast to get treatments every two weeks. He said that it would be hard during Covid restrictions but that it could be done.

I talked to Ben and told him that my treatment was canceled again, and he said to come home. He said that he would fly in as scheduled and that we could drive back home together. We made the plan.

I told Michelle our plans, and she thought that I might be leaving because of their fighting. I assured her that was not the reason, and I thanked her for letting me stay for as long as I did. I hoped that I was helpful with fixing up the apartment and knew that she needed to rent it out now and get some additional income coming in.

I was concerned, of course about how I was going to travel from Prescott to Washington DC in the middle of a pandemic, but I would take up that issue when the time came.

Ben flew in, and I picked him up at the airport. We spent a day with Michelle and Mark, packed up the Audi and headed for home. I still had the Bells' Palsy bad, and I was glad that Ben was with me to help me with the drive this time. He did almost all the driving. I finally decided to give him a break, and we hit a detour on the Interstate, which took us onto some backroads. There had been some freezing rain and snow forecast for that day, but it was supposed to be exceptionally light. Well, the road that I was on quickly became quite hazardous. Not only was I plagued with a bad eye, but now I had to drive on a sheet of ice for what seemed like forever. Ben told me to pull over, but that was a problem because the road was so narrow. I was driving in ruts that had been made by a large semi ahead of me in the opposite lane. I did not feel comfortable driving out of those tire tracks. I was also afraid to stop in the middle of the road since visibility was poor, so I kept driving. I white-knuckled it for about three hours before finally pulling over to let Ben drive.

Of course, as soon as he got behind the wheel, the roads began to improve. The rest of the drive was uneventful, and after three days, we pulled into my driveway in Prescott. To my complete surprise, the entire front yard was decorated with yellow ribbons on all the trees, and there was a big gold sign that read WELCOME HOME on my garage doors. We parked in the garage, and my dogs greeted me with mixed emotions. Deedee cried and cried and jumped all over me while Pita went to Ben and kept his distance from me. He was curious for sure, but he did not come to me right away. I had to go to him, and he was giving me a little cold shoulder. I already knew that he would be this way. Anytime I left home, it was the same. He was punishing me for leaving him. He eventually came around and then would not leave my side.

It was so great to be home. I got caught up on a dental cleaning and saw an ophthalmologist for my eyesight. Between the Bell's Palsy and the chemo, I could not drive at night any longer, and it was getting harder and harder to see the signs on the roads from any distance. The eye exam confirmed that I had cataracts, so I scheduled that surgery, hoping that my Bell's Palsy would resolve by then. I told everyone that asked me how I was doing that even with the facial paralysis and other side effects that immunotherapy was nowhere near as bad as chemo or radiation.

"Live with intention. Walk to the edge. Listen hard. Practice wellness. Play with abandon. Laugh. Choose without regret. Appreciate. Continue to learn. Do what you love. Live as if this is all there is. "

Anna Pereira

Chapter 27

Freedom

I was due for another visit to NIH on the 21st and 22nd of December. Unfortunately, it was scan time again. I wished that I could have gotten the vaccine before this trip, but I would once again have to mask up for travel. The good news is that hardly anyone was traveling. The bad news was that I would now have to stay masked on a plane for 5.5 hours each way, and I would have to stay three nights instead of two.

My travel dates came around quickly, and I took off for DC. I had to fly in on Sunday. I had my blood tests and scans done on Monday. Tuesday, I would get my results and treatment, and then Wednesday, I would fly home. My Bell's Palsy was still active, although it was much better. I wondered if they might withhold treatment again.

The travel, labs, and scans went smoothly, and on Tuesday morning, while waiting in the clinic for the nurse to set up our zoom call, I experienced a tinge of fear. This scan, according to Strauss, was going to tell me much more than my first one. If the treatments were not working, they would have that news for me today. I wondered how I would handle it if the news was bad. I had no one with me to lean on. I thought to myself; I can do this.

We said our hellos over the zoom call, and I could hear Dr. Strauss's kids in the background. They sounded incredibly young. He apologized for the interruption, and I told him that it was no problem.

"They are probably excited about the upcoming holidays," I said.

"Yes," he said. "They are non-stop."

"Your blood tests look pretty good," he began.

"Can you address the more pressing news," I asked?

"Sure," he laughed. Your scans are clear!"

"Wait, what?" I asked.

"The treatment is working,"

I started to cry happy tears.

"Really?" I asked him. "Are you saying that you see no more enlarged lymph nodes and no spots?"

"I am saying exactly that."

The nurse and the other doctor in the room both congratulated me. Dr. Strauss then said that I would be taken off the drugs. He said that there was no reason to give them to me at this point and that it would only aggravate my Bell's Palsy. He called me one of his early graduates and told me that I would be helping a lot of people. I cried again. What a Christmas present, I thought to myself.

The rest of the visit was quite surreal. I couldn't believe what my ears were hearing.

I thanked them all, and then I said, "I don't even want to ask what would happen if it comes back because I want to believe that I have been cured. I just need to know if the treatments will be available to me in the future."

Dr. Strauss assured me that they would. He told me that I was technically still in the trial and recommended that I scan again in three to six months. I told him the six months sounded good, and he thought for a minute and then said that he liked the three months just a tad better. I agreed. Dr. Strauss said that I could have them done at Mayo if I liked. I felt like he was my guardian angel. I would have given him a big hug, but it was Covid, and he was on video. I think I must have thanked him another ten times before we closed the call.

Because treatment was canceled, I had the whole afternoon. I called Ben, Michelle, and Tony with the exciting news before leaving the hospital. They were ecstatic. Later, I texted everyone that was staying connected with me regularly. Many commented that this news had just made their day. I told the cab driver and the Starbucks cashier. I wanted to scream it from the rooftop of my hotel. One thing I didn't do was to post it on my Anal Cancer Group site, at least not yet. I eventually would, but it's so hard. I wanted all of us to have good news, but life is not fair. I knew it would be important for those newly diagnosed and for those with metastatic disease to see others surviving. I needed to tell them the details of my trial. There would be many questions from the group about which therapies I was on. Many have been told that standard protocols are no longer working. They need to know that they have some new hope. I am also aware that most won't consider participating in a clinical trial. I don't fully understand it but they obviously have their reasons.

First off, why do doctors even say that a patient is out of options? A survivor on our site once mentioned that her doctor said that they were out of options and that she had six months to a year left. He told her that she should enjoy the rest of her days. She went to see Dr. Cathy Eng at Vanderbilt at the instruction of another survivor in our group, and Dr. Eng told her that she had a lot more options. She tried a couple of different protocols and then finally found one that stabilized the woman's UG. Over three years later, she is still alive. I would make sure to post my success story before I turned in for the night. If I can help even one person, it will be my honor.

I was hungry, so I decided to treat myself to an indulgent dinner. I ordered and picked up a gyros sandwich, French fries, and a piece of Baklava cheesecake for dinner. I decided that I needed a beer to go with that, so I went down to the lobby. The bar was closed, of course, so I ordered it from the receptionist. She was having a hard time finding an opener for my Corona, and she called the manager to help her look. I told him that I was celebrating because my scans came back clear today. He was so happy for me; he said that the beer was on him, and did I want two? I said thank you so much, but that one would be plenty.

After returning home, I went through my days with a new appreciation for life. I was so grateful for my response to the treatments. Not everyone gets this opportunity. I looked at every little thing as a gift. I noticed and appreciated so much more than I ever had before; in nature, in myself, and in others.

I had heard about an old Irish custom to welcome in the new year. It is said that you must open your door at exactly midnight and let the old year out and welcome the new year in. I'm not Irish, but it seemed like the perfect thing to do this New Year's Eve. I set my alarm clock, woke up, and opened every door in my house that evening. I said goodbye to the last two years of my life. I was more than ready for a new beginning.

I spent the following months in a great mood. If anyone asked how I was doing, my answer was "fantastic." I started golfing more often and got my vaccine when it was my turn. Well, I got it a bit early. I found out that if you volunteered at the hospital, you could get your shots early. So, I signed up to volunteer and liked it so much; I went back two more times. All I really did was help the line move along, and if someone needed a wheelchair, I wheeled them in. I enjoyed chatting with the people and helped ease their hesitancy in many cases by telling them how easy it was. It amazed me how many people are afraid of a needle. I called myself a human pin cushion as a joke.

I added some of my supplements back into my routine. The first being the AHCC. After that, I continued with the pre and probiotics. I decided to hold off on the IV therapy because Dr. Strauss told me to be careful with overstimulation of my immune system right now.

It began slowly in Chicago, and then I really started noticing it during the winter of 2021. I started to put my weight back on. After returning from Chicago, I weighed myself, and I had gained five pounds. I was up to 115, and I felt stronger. By the end of February, I weighed in at a whopping 121 pounds. I never thought I would gain weight again, but now it was coming back on at a steady pace. I figured that I was finally absorbing my nutrients better. I maintained a strict diet except for sourdough bread. A new bakery opened in town, and they had the best organic sourdough bread. I know that sourdough is a little better for me than regular bread, but it is still wheat, and wheat turns to glucose. I learned that if you are going to cheat a little on your diet, you should exercise right after you eat. Then the glucose gets used as an energy source. A little protein with those carbs is also an excellent choice as the protein helps you to build muscle. For this to work best, you also need to drink plenty of fluids. So, if I cheat, exercise is my punishment.

My next scans were done at Mayo, and I was excited to see Dr. Jordan and Jackie again. I brought each of them a small gift. I started to needle-felt soap bars. I would make the soaps into round bars and then use a hot and icy water method with friction, rubbing to cover it with roving wool. I would then use more wool in assorted colors to make designs in the wool. You do this with needles that have very tiny hooks on the end of them. These are called felted soaps. They are beautiful, and I have gotten pretty good at making them. A felted soap bar is like soap and loofah in one. I handed them their felted soaps, and they had no idea what they were, so I had to explain. I made a beautiful lilac-scented shea butter soap covered in yellow with bright pink and purple flowers for Jackie. For Dr. Jordan, I made a goat's milk bar scented with sandalwood and cypress. It was a neutral tan with brown snowcapped mountains, pine trees, and a big orange setting sun. After greeting one another and presenting their gifts, I straightened up and prepared myself for the results. Dr. Jordan got right to it and said my scans were completely clear. This setting was where I had gotten the worst news of my life, and now finally, the tides had turned. They thanked me for their gifts, and I thanked them for always taking such good care of me and apologized for being a pain in the butt at times. I explained that Dr. Strauss wanted me to scan every three months and that I might see them again in a few.

Mayo sent the scans to NIH, and a few days later, I spoke with Dr. Strauss. I wanted confirmation from him that the radiologists at NIH agreed, and he confirmed that the scans were indeed clear. I thanked him repeatedly and asked him how the other patients were doing. I wanted to know if I was the only one. He told me that I was one of just two patients with complete remission. There were fourteen of us in the trial currently, and he told me that the others were also doing quite well. He said that their scans showed stability and some shrinkage. He told me that the M7824 now had a name. It is called Bintrafusp Alfa. I told him that I would likely always call it by its number. He said that trials for other cancers did not go as well as those for HPV cancers. For some reason, the HPV cancer responded much better. He reminded me that he would like another follow-up scan in three months and not to be a stranger. He told me to feel free to text or email him whenever.

The baby boomers were now almost all fully vaccinated. It felt so much better to know that my husband and all our neighbors and buddies now had protection. Saturday Night Live had a great sketch called *Boomers Got the Vax*. It's hilarious. We were all out and about, having a good old time, and the young ones had to quarantine. That's very close to how it was in the real world.

I decided to make an appointment with Dr. Zander and tell him the good news. I also needed to start back on a prevention protocol. We had a Telehealth call, and he was thrilled for me. He said that I was amazing and that I should not doubt that all the added protocols I had taken had a lot to do with my success. He felt that it kept my UG small.

Dr. Zander said, "When the immunotherapy hit it, it was already weakened and didn't have a chance."

He felt very strongly about my starting TM at this stage, and I told him that I remember talking about this with Dr. Rubin after my first line of conventional treatments, but I was too sick to consider it back then. He sent me some more information on it, and I said that I would look into it. TM stands for tetrathiomolybdate, a copper chelator. Studies have determined that copper is an important cofactor for angiogenesis.[xxx] Dr. Zander told me that it could help prevent another recurrence but that I would have to get regular blood tests to keep the level exactly right.

I'm fairly sure that Dr. Strauss will have an issue with my taking this since I am technically still in the trial until September 1st. I will keep that in my back pocket along with several other UG-fighting strategies. I have learned much from my research and from others who are passionate about finding a cure.

During my research, I came across studies being done with gene editing. This is amazing and so futuristic. If only it can be harnessed and used for only good-intentioned purposes. It is molecular biology at its finest. It is based on a simplified version of the bacterial CRISPR-Cas9 antiviral defense system. An enzyme can modify DNA. I know that this virus has damaged our DNA, so maybe soon we will be able to fix it. Recent studies have shown progress against the herpes virus and HPV. In HPV, the gene-editing targets E6 and E7 proteins. Remember those? In animal studies, tumors have been eliminated. These studies are very recent and ongoing. It's more reason not to give up.

My heart goes out to those that have suffered and are still suffering. It is, without doubt, a complicated disease, and we should be throwing everything at it. I know that I am most fortunate to be able to afford the alternative treatments that I discussed in this book, but I think that even those of you who have limited funds can do much to contribute to your health. The Budwig protocol is very inexpensive. Juicing is not costly. A mostly vegan diet can be easily achieved. Seeing an Integrative Oncologist as a second opinion is often covered by insurance, as they are MD's. Immunotherapy drugs are now available for many UGs. If not for your UG, then seek out a clinical trial. These trials are low cost or completely free in many cases. Special requests can be made to the drug manufacturers (keep bugging them) and there is always the Social Medwork in Amsterdam. Off-label drugs are very inexpensive. Find a doctor who will prescribe them for you. They are out there. Join support groups where other survivors can help you find what you need. We are more than willing to help. I have witnessed survivors sharing recipes, protocols, books, rides, equipment, physician referrals and more.

Our healthcare system is nowhere near perfect but it is all we have. Take comfort knowing that the new UG drugs are much safer than current therapies. There are scientists, immunologists, biologists and physicians that are dedicating their lives to finding a cure. I have no doubt that we are closer than ever. Physicians are starting to understand that many of their patients want more than just to address their symptoms. They want to address the causes of their illnesses. Precision medicine offers customized care through the use of genetic testing. New immunotherapy drugs are harnessing the power of our immune systems. New epigenetic drugs are being researched and may turn our UG cells back to normal instead of destroying them. Scientists are learning more about the pathways that drive metastasis and are working to prevent growth. We want solutions that work with our bodies natural defense mechanisms. Our immune systems are powerful and efficient when they are working optimally. Do not assume that an advanced UG diagnosis is a death sentence. This is not necessarily the case anymore.

"May you be at peace. May your heart remain open. May you awaken to the light of your own true nature. May you be healed. May you be a source of healing for all beings."

Tibetan Buddhist Prayer

Chapter 28

Forward

I went on to get another clear scan in June and again in September. I don't know what the future will hold for me, but I am super grateful. I want to dedicate the rest of my life to helping others overcome advanced UG. That's why I wrote this book. I am now two years post treatment and I just got accepted as a mentor for newly diagnosed Anal UG patients. I look forward to helping them. My next venture will be to start a support group for advanced UG patients in my home town.

I am traveling more and hitting some items on my bucket list. Not because I am worried about dying but because there is no time like the present. I have always wanted to play in the World Series of Poker in Las Vegas. The Ladies event is a four-day Texas Hold 'Em tournament, if you make it that far. The winner gets a wad of cash and a Champion Bracelet. I signed up and there were 644 participants. In order to "cash" you have to make it to number 97. We started out with 72 tables and I actually made it to the final six tables and came in 51st place! It was an absolute blast! I am making plans to renew my wedding vows and have the big reception party that I never had with my second marriage. No more regrets! I have perfected my felted soaps to darling animals. They all have tails and I am going to call them Tails Felted Soaps and start and Etsy shop where I will sell them and send the profits to the Anal Cancer Foundation. I am hoping to recruit other survivors to help me felt them.

In October I received some news that caused me a great deal of concern. Dr. Strauss called me and told me that the Bintrafusp Alfa (M7824) might be taken out of clinical trials and might not be available to us in the future. He said that the committee recommended to discontinue all production because in the Lung and Biliary Tract Cancer Trials it had not helped patients and had actually made things worse for them. He told me that for some reason however, it was working with HPV cancers only, including Cervical and Head and Neck Cancers. I did not understand why they would want to take this away from us since so many patients were benefitting. I guess it is about money or numbers in the end. He suggested I write a letter to them explaining my personal story. He said that this sometimes helps. This was my letter:

I am writing this letter with a heavy heart. I was just recently informed that you are considering pulling Bintrafusp Alfa (M7824) from all clinical trials due to its ineffectiveness in lung and biliary tract cancers. While this may be true, it is not true for HPV cancers, especially in the combination trial that includes IL12 and the PDS 101 HPV vaccine. I hope that my story will convince you of it's value and effectiveness.

In January of 2019 at 59 years of age, I was diagnosed with stage 3C anal cancer. Like many others, I was misdiagnosed as having hemorrhoids for a year before finally discovering the 7cm tumor and involvement of several pelvic lymph nodes. My odds for a cure were grim and Dr. Ashman, my Radiation Oncologist at Mayo in Scottsdale said that he would have to "hit it hard!" Treatment for Anal Cancer has remained virtually the same for the last 40 years. They were advising the Nigro Protocol which consists of 30 days of pelvic radiation (54 gy), which would leave me with devastating lifelong side-effects. I would also be getting two of the oldest and strongest chemotherapeutics on the market, Mitomycin and Flouroracil (Five FU). I was to receive 200 hours of chemo in just 8 days. I searched high and low to find any other alternative to this protocol. This is when I first came in contact with Dr. Strauss at NIH. He told me that I could get into the M7824 trial but I would have to turn down chemoradiation and he advised me strongly against that. He said that if my cancer came back and he hoped that it would not, that he could then get me into the trial.

I started chemoradiation in April of 2019 and by May I had lost over 30 pounds, had two trips to the ER for dehydration and chest pain and got a horrific rash all over my body. For the next six months, I was in and out of the ER another 4 times, lost another 20 pounds and had severe chest pain and debilitating fatigue on a daily basis. I went into a complete depression and was diagnosed with PTSD which prevented me from entering the Nivolumab trial which I needed to begin within two months of my treatment. My first set of scans were clear and I finally turned the corner and started to maintain my weight in October of 2019. By my next set of scans in January, my team started to see signs of possible metastases. In March of 2020, it was confirmed that my cancer had metastasized to my para aortic lymph nodes and to my lungs. My doctors at Mayo then recommended Nivolumab since the chemotherapy did not work for me.

Before agreeing to the Nivolumab, I decided to contact Dr. Strauss again and he said that he was sorry that my cancer came back. He then told me about a new trial that had just started with a combination of three biologics. The M7824, IL12 and an HPV vaccine. He said that they hoped this would be a better option than the Nivolumab for patients like myself. He told me that the first set of patients had to have some side effects resolved before he could enroll any new patients and that I might have to wait a couple of months for that to happen. After speaking with my team, they agreed that I could wait as long as my back pain did not get worse. I was having pain and numbness in my back and legs anytime I walked more than a block or two. They admitted that the combination trials were offering more promise than the checkpoint inhibitors on their own. I decided to wait for the trial and began in September of 2020, during the peak of Covid. After just two treatments, the pain in my back and legs subsided. I knew that it was working. The first time I took the full combination, I got the chills and fever so bad that I had to change my clothes and sheets five times in one night. I felt certain that it had jolted my immune system into a high gear. I got side effects like increased rectal bleeding and even an episode of Bell's Palsy but it was still 100 times better than chemotherapy. I missed a couple of doses because of the Bell's Palsy. In spite of those missed doses, Dr. Strauss was feeling optimistic after my first scan and after just four months and four treatments, my second scan showed I was in remission. The spots on my lungs were gone! My lymph nodes were smaller and they were now saying that I could stop the treatments and just come back for follow up scans every three months. OMG! It was the best Christmas present ever. I had only one question. I asked if the drug combo would be available to me if I needed it in the future and my team at NIH felt certain that it would be. It now had a name. It was called Bitrafusp Alfa. That made me feel confident that this combination could also help others like me in the future. Dr. Strauss said that the other patients with HPV cancers were also benefitting from the combination trial. He said that they lowered the dose of the IL12 to half the dose that I took. I put myself out there with a brand new set of biologics to establish correct dosing and monitor side effects. I traveled every two weeks during a pandemic with a compromised immune system. I felt proud and humbled that I could be of some service to future patients diagnosed with this awful stigmatized cancer. I wanted to shout it to the world. I wrote a book and called it "HINDsight in 2020". In my book, I talk about my life and my cancer journey during the pandemic. My story culminates with the clinical trial that saved my life.

Anal Cancer is now growing at a staggering 3 percent per year. With over 80% of the population now living with HPV, this is no surprise. I don't know what the statistics are for Cervical or Head and Neck Cancers but I do know that this combination helped those patients as well. I know that we are not a huge group but we do represent 5% of all cancers and I think that more oncologists should be aware of these trials. If others knew about the trials, more patients would enroll. I had to find them on my own. I have been posting my progress on several Facebook cancer groups. Many advanced anal cancer patients simply follow the guidance of their oncologists who are still treating them with chemotherapy. They know nothing about this trial.

I have now gained back half the weight I lost from chemo and my energy levels are almost back to normal. I appreciate every day of my life with my three children and three grandchildren. I get a bit of anxiety every three months when I have to rescan but knowing that these drugs are available to me if I need them helps to keep me grounded. Please don't discontinue the trials with this very remarkable life-saving drug, especially the combination trial. Our lives are depending on them.

Thank you for your consideration.

Sincerely,

Elaine Bonney
Stage 4 Anal Cancer Survivor

Merck KGAA, the maker of the drug decided to continue the combination trail and keep supplying the drug, before I even had a chance to send my letter. There were several patients trying to reach them and the Anal Cancer Foundation also got involved. I think all of this helped to convince them not to pull it from production. I understand that they are even planning to start some additional combination trials. I plan to send my letter anyway.

My side effects from chemo, radiation, and immunotherapy remain with me as a reminder of all I have been through. I have more fatigue, for sure. I finally got an echocardiogram to look at any potential damage to my heart. It is minimal but there is some mild mitral valve regurgitation which is likely causing my fatigue. I am going to assume that my body will work to heal this. I have some pelvic bone pain and just had a bone density test done. I have osteoporosis of the lower vertebrae. I plan to take supplements to avoid future fractures. I continue to have mild rectal bleeding from fissures, and I will treat this with ozone if it gets worse. I have occasional intestinal issues that I control with my diet. Pelvic floor therapy is something that I will look into if this gets worse. My vagina is atrophied, and the skin is extremely delicate. I am addressing these issues with DHEA and Estrogen pellets, but I have to closely monitor my blood hormone levels because too much is carcinogenic. Finally, the left side of my face is somewhat slanted, and my eyesight is a bit blurred from Bell's Palsy. I wear that as just another battle scar.

As a survivor, change is everything. Through my journey, I have learned how to make those changes in my life. I know now that what I think, feel, and believe has a profound effect on my world.

When I was at the lowest point in my life, I thought I was being punished. I felt that I deserved my disease and I believed that I would die from it. I looked back at the people and circumstances that formed my personality and I realized that I could learn from those moments. I forgave myself for my past mistakes. How could I blame the little girl that grew up without a mother and in an era where she knew nothing about the dangers of drugs or unprotected sex?

I still have my dreams of flying, but they are different now. I soar higher and with greater ease. While there are still dangers below me, I no longer fear them like I once did.

"She stood in the storm, and when the wind did not blow her way, she adjusted her sails."

Anonymous

Epilogue

I want to thank you for reading my story. Many of the quotes that you see at the end of each chapter have come from the Facebook page of a friend and fellow golfer who recently died from Cervical Cancer. These were hand-picked by her as she valiantly fought for her life. I just wanted to honor her in some small way.

Additionally, I am excited because I just saw that the NCCN has just put out a guideline for Anal Cancer patients. *Wow!* Now this is progress. With support from the Anal Cancer Foundation and endorsed by the HPV Alliance (co-founded by Marcia Cross), the guide provides newly diagnosed patients with most of the information they may need to make educated decisions about their treatment options. This essential guide includes Risk Factors, Diagnosis and Treatment Planning, Staging, Questions to Ask your Doctor, Fertility and Family Planning, Follow-up and Surveillance, Recurrence, Metastatic Anal Cancer, Clinical Trial Information, and Management of Late and Long-Term Side Effects. All I can say is that it is about time!

Anal Cancer and HPV Resources:

NCCN.org/patients

Analcancerfoundation.org

HPVAlliance.com

Additional Resources for All cancer patients:

The American Cancer Society http://www.cancer.org

National Institute of Health

http://www.ncbi.nlm.nih.gov fax line 01-402-5874

The American Board of Medical Specialties

http://www.abms.org

The American Medical Association

http://www.ama-assn.org

Center for Alternative Medicine Research in Cancer

http://www.sph.uth.tmc.edu/utcam

Facebook Groups mentioned in this book:

SQ1 Support Group

AnalCancer Support

Know More: AnalCancer

Clinical Trials-Anal Cancer

Jane McLelland Off-Label Drugs for Cancer

You Me, and Immunotherapy

Recap For Those Newly Diagnosed with Anal Cancer

This part of my book can act as a quick reference guide for you. If you have been recently diagnosed, you may feel pressure to start treatment, and I want you to have this critical information at hand. Remember to breathe and try not to get too overwhelmed. It is a lot to take in. Just take it one step at a time.

While still considered rare, Anal Cancer is now the fastest-growing cancer in the United States, increasing at a staggering 3% per year. A high-risk HPV virus causes over ninety percent of Anal Cancers. There is now a way to prevent HPV in our children and young adults. A vaccine (Gardasil-9 by Merck) is available for those between the ages of 11 and 45. It is approved up to age 45 and recommended up to age 26 for both men and women. It protects against several strains of HPV including those that cause cancer. Ask your primary care physician. It is best to get this vaccine series before sexual activity.

There are over 100 strains of HPV virus, and only a few cause cancer. HPV is an STD. You do not have to have anal sex to get Anal Cancer. In fact, you do not have to have intercourse at all. It is from skin-to-skin contact. Most people get it during sexual activities. Nearly 85% of adults between the ages of 18 and 65 have at least one strain of HPV. It is the most common sexually transmitted infection. It is estimated that 80 million people carry this virus and most do not have symptoms. HPV can lie dormant in your body for decades. If you have had several partners, there is no way to tell who gave it to you. Having more sexual partners increases your chances.

Anal Cancer is still exceedingly rare, and most people that have HPV will NOT get cancer. Their immune systems usually fight it off or keep it at bay. Most Anal Cancer patients are female (about two-thirds). The average age at diagnosis is 59. It is very similar to Cervical Cancer. It is quite different from Colorectal Cancer. Still, it is technically considered a subcategory of Colorectal Cancer at health institutions.

HPV can cause warts, but warts can also be caused by the Herpes virus. These can be genital warts, or they can appear on other areas of your body. You can have many strains of HPV simultaneously. Having more than one strain of HPV or having herpes with it can increase your chances of getting cancer, but you must also have the deadly strain, like HPV 16 or 18. If you take a test for HPV, it is not always accurate. It often comes out as a false negative when the virus is not currently active. If you have HPV, recurring warts, or have had a pap smear showing precancerous cells, you should be on guard. Avoid touching warts. HPV is spread by skin to skin contact. Keep warts dry. Do not engage in sex acts when genital warts are present.

You should get pap smears more often, and you should get a DRE (digital rectal exam) from your primary care physician or gynecologist every year or two. Tell your doctor that you want this. Very few doctors will check your anal canal, but they should if you already have HPV or precancerous cells. You can ask for an anal pap smear if you have rectal bleeding and/or any feeling of blockage or any lesion outside of your anus. You should also get a colonoscopy every five years, starting at age 45. Make sure you tell the doctor to look for Anal Cancer because they often miss it or diagnose it as hemorrhoids. Please don't allow them to cut into anything on your first colonoscopy, and make sure a reputable gastroenterologist or colorectal surgeon does it. I have heard from far too many Anal Cancer patients who were first diagnosed with hemorrhoids by mistake, even after a colonoscopy. Some doctors have attempted to remove the hemorrhoid only to find out that it is cancerous after the fact. You only want a colorectal surgeon to remove your tumor and only if it is very small. If you have rectal bleeding, do not assume it is hemorrhoids, even if your doctor says it is. Take it seriously and get an anal pap smear, colonoscopy, HRA (high-resolution anoscopy), or sigmoidoscopy. If you have an external lesion, do not assume it is a hemorrhoid. Anal Cancer can grow inside or outside the anus, or both. Anal Cancer can start as AIN (anal intraepithelial neoplasia). These are precancerous anal lesions that can very easily turn cancerous and must not be confused with hemorrhoids.

If, after a biopsy, you are diagnosed with Anal Cancer, do not blame yourself or your partner. You did absolutely nothing to deserve it.

You are going to need to make some particularly important decisions. I advise you to take all the stress out of your life. Do it now by repairing all strained relationships and forgiving all enemies. Nothing is worth the stress any longer; your body cannot take it. You must have a clear mind. If you are used to taking care of others, stop and get help if you can. This is the time to take care of "you." What good will you be to anyone else if you do not get through this? Love yourself and take care of yourself. Accept help if it is offered. Ask for the help you need.

A biopsy of your tumor can identify if your cancer is Squamous Cell or Adenocarcinoma and HPV positive. It can also tell you how fast your cells are dividing or growing. I am not convinced that a biopsy is your best choice when the tumor is small and not already bleeding. Many reputable physicians now believe that opening a lesion can allow it to spread. Do your own research on this. In retrospect, I would not have allowed a biopsy at the time of my colonoscopy. I would have had an anoscopy or sigmoidoscopy done by a qualified colorectal surgeon if my GI suspected Anal Cancer after a colonoscopy. With a sigmoidoscopy, you will get to see the lesion yourself, and you will get a very good measurement of its size. A surgeon can also palpate some of your pelvic lymph nodes to see if they are enlarged. In my opinion, you would then have more time to treat it alternatively if it is small and if this is of interest to you. If you treat it alternatively, you must get blood tests and scans to ensure that it is not growing. If you must have a biopsy, then get it done. I would also have genetic testing done on my tumor and blood. An RGCC test can tell you which immunotherapies and chemotherapies will work for you specifically and which supplements and herbs can benefit you.

Most oncologists have zero experience with Anal Cancer. It is rare. Even if you love your doctor, it is no substitute for experience! They are not gods. Get two or even three opinions, and make sure that you look for an oncologist with experience. We get three quotes on a car repair, but we trust only one doctor with our lives. That seems counter-intuitive. You may have to travel to find this person or team. It often takes a team. Your team should consist of a Radiation Oncologist, a Medical Oncologist, and a Colorectal Surgeon. You will also need a Gastroenterologist on hand, and I strongly recommend a Naturopath and Integrative doctor specializing in oncology. Most insurance will not pay for the services of a naturopath, but all the others should be covered. Do this in every case, but especially in advanced cases and when you are advised an APR. Surgery can save your life, but please make sure that it is necessary before you do it. Serious complications can arise if it is not done properly. This could mean a lifelong stoma, serious infection, or worse. In some emergency cases, a surgeon may need to do an APR that is later reversed. Ask if a reversal is possible if it is not offered.

Some of the institutions that treat Anal Cancer patients are MD Anderson, Memorial Sloan Kettering, Moffit, Vanderbilt Medical Center, and others. Unfortunately, even at the facilities just mentioned, most oncologists are limited in their knowledge and will advise only the NCCN standard of care protocols, which can be dated. Ask your oncologist for the recently published *NCCN Guideline for Anal Cancer Patients*.

If you decide to get the conventional treatment, the odds are in your favor that you will be cured. Cured in medical terminology means that you will survive at least five years. After two years cancer free, your odds go up. After you make your treatment decision, you must embrace it and believe that it will cure you! Believe this as strongly as you can.

The current standard of care is chemo-radiation. This treatment is known as the Nigro protocol and is currently advised for most stages of Anal Cancer. Cancer treatments are always changing, so make sure you know the very latest in treatment options. You will have to do your own research. Don't assume your oncologist will do this for you. Some stage 1 and stage 2A patients can have theirs surgically removed. You will probably be treated with the Nigro protocol if it is a larger tumor or has any lymph node involvement. If you are at a very advanced stage, you may be given higher doses of radiation and a stronger combination of chemotherapy drugs. This is especially important. If you have advanced Anal Cancer, in addition to getting two or three competent opinions, I also suggest you investigate current clinical trials. Your targeted genomic test can help you to understand which new drugs can offer you the best outcome.

In most cases, your oncologist will not do this for you. They may even tell you that there are no current trials. You need to research this yourself or get someone you trust to do it for you. It is easy. The website is clinicaltrials.gov, and you can search Anal Cancer. I also searched HPV cancers so that I did not miss anything. I limited my search to the United States, but there are trials all over the world. Once you find and narrow down the trials as much as possible, show them to your team. They can help you determine if you are a candidate or not. You can also call or email the lead investigator listed for the trial. Some trials are available as a first-line treatment, and you should check those out in advance. Even if I had a small tumor, I would look into this before proceeding with surgery or treatment. Most of these trials now involve Immunotherapeutics. This is the wave of the future.

Immunotherapy works with your own immune system and helps it to recognize your cancer and kill it. It is much less toxic to your body than chemo and/or radiation. Very soon, chemotherapy and radiation will be replaced by other treatments, primarily Immunotherapy. These will replace current first-line treatments for cancers. Many experts believe this to be true. That is why so much money is being thrown at research for these new classes of drugs. We are at the forefront of an exciting turn for the better in cancer treatment. An Immunologist will want the results from your genetic testing and will know how to interpret them.

Nigro (a forty-year-old protocol) depends heavily on radiation in that it does most of the work. Chemo is just there to mop up what may be left over. I had 30 radiation treatments to my pelvic area, and I believe this to be standard. Look up 'The NCCN guidelines for Anal Cancer.' These are primarily for healthcare professionals but they are available to you online. Radiation is given consecutively or every weekday for six weeks. It is not advisable to miss a treatment, but you may have to for various reasons. I found out after the fact that it is best to get your radiation treatments as late in the day as possible or in the evening if it is offered when your circadian rhythm is winding down. They will radiate most of your lymph nodes in this area even if they see your cancer only in one node to ensure they get any microscopic spread. Your radiation oncologists and other radiologists map out these radiation treatments to avoid your vital organs and hit just the tumor and lymph nodes. There are currently three types of radiation that are used for Anal Cancer that I know of. Most use IMRT (intensity modulated radiation therapy).[xxxi] IMPT (intensity modulated proton therapy) is a newer approach not currently paid for by insurance but may be available. Another uses Two-Dimensional Photon Therapy or "Conventional Radiation Therapy." If your hospital only offers this, you may want to look elsewhere for the newer treatments. You will want IMPT or IMRT to lessen the side effects. If your insurance won't pay for IMPT, you may be able to get it within the context of a clinical trial. I understand that they are similar in effectiveness against the cancer. The difference is with side effects. You should know all the possible side effects from your radiation and prepare your body in advance for this barrage. Some hospitals are now using vaginal dilators during radiation. At the very least, you should be starting them two weeks post-treatment.

You should take part in your healing process. Even if your oncologist tells you otherwise, there are things you can do to prevent serious side effects such as GI issues, Lymphedema and Neuropathy, just to name a few. You can also increase your odds of success by implementing a multi-modal approach. According to William Faloon, co-Founder of the Life Extension Foundation, alternative therapies can play an important role not only in mitigating side effects from conventional treatments, but also in suppressing survival factors that enable cancer cells to escape destruction.

My protocol used two very potent chemotherapeutic agents. They are Mitomycin and Fluorouracil (Five FU). Some patients have been treated with Cisplatin and Five FU (usually in more advanced cases). Most are treated with Mitomycin and Capecitabine (an oral chemo pill). Capecitabine can cause hand-foot syndrome and will likely be stopped if there is evidence of this side effect. There are also some newer chemotherapy agents being used, and sometimes these may be offered orally. Usually, this will be in the context of a trial and for lower stages. It will take you five or six weeks to complete the treatment plan. The Mitomycin is given by IV push on day one and day 21. The Five FU is also given on days 1 and 21, but you will get a chemo bag that is attached to you through a PICC line or port, and it drips into you slowly for over 96 hours each round. You should ask for a test in advance to ensure that your body contains the DPD enzyme, which is necessary to process 5-FU. You could die if you do not have this enzyme.

If you have chest pain, do not assume it is heartburn. Five-FU can cause dilated cardiomyopathy. This is a disease where your heart muscle becomes weak and doesn't pump blood to the rest of the body as well as it should. This may not show up on an EKG or in blood tests. Have a cardiologist do an echocardiogram. The infused or drip method for administration of Five-FU is worse on your heart muscle than the Bolus or oral delivery. Make sure you know exactly how much anti-nausea medication to take and when to take them. Do not get nauseous or sick first, or you may not be able to keep the pills down or keep hydrated. Ensure you know all your possible side effects from the chemo and what to do if you get them. Before you start chemotherapy, make sure that you get your body ready for it. Your Naturopathic Oncologist or

Integrative Oncologist can help you with a plan. You need to drink a ton of water before, during, and after chemo. I mean, drown yourself with clean, pure water. Also, consider fasting right before you start. Studies show you will not get as sick, and it will work better.

Most of the support you get from your oncologists will center around healing from radiation burns. These burns are visible and painful. You will be given pain meds and salves. Use them until your burns are healed. Chemo can also cause a great deal of distress in your body. They won't talk about this as much. It will target and kill all your fast-growing cells, and your GI tract is full of those cells (from your mouth down to your rectum). It can cause extreme fatigue and Neutropenia (a serious drop in white blood cell counts). Radiation will cause you late side effects, including extreme fatigue, GI issues such as diarrhea, frequent gas, urgency, stress fractures, and vaginal atrophy. There are medications, supplements, therapy, and diet changes that can help tremendously. Hyperbaric oxygen treatments and pelvic floor exercises can also help.

Your healing process is not just physical. It may very well include healing spiritually or psychologically. Get help if you are depressed. Let your feelings out, but if your anxiety and depression persist for too long, it can seriously affect your physical health. Consider EMDR for unresolved trauma. I strongly recommend that you embrace the mind-body connection. It is very real. Your mind is enormously powerful. You need to believe that your body is healing. Learn to meditate and embrace positive energy practices daily. Consider meditation, Reiki, and acupuncture to help with energy flow. Surround yourself with supportive people, and don't get annoyed by those that are unsupportive. They are simply incapable.

Once you get through recovery, do not go back to your old ways. Let me repeat, do not go back to your old ways. Keep active and follow an anti-cancer diet. It's not about absolute abstention. Consider a water fast every so often to boost your immune system. Keep your cancer from growing again by keeping it weak. Don't give it what it needs to grow. Practice a positive attitude. Keep up on your scans. This cancer could come back. I don't want to scare you, but you won't change permanently if you don't keep realistic.

Keep on a supplement regimen to hold your HPV virus down. Medicinal mushrooms can help with this. I use AHCC and a liquid tincture from my Naturopath, and I am unsure exactly what they do, but I don't get warts when I am on them. Somehow, they work with my immune system to keep herpes and/or HPV at bay. Ongoing clinical trials confirm this.

Keep exploring ways to prevent metastases with your Naturopath or Integrative doctors. There are many new privately funded trials going on for exciting new alternative methods. Don't dismiss this as quackery—patients who add alternative treatments to their conventional treatments live longer.

It probably won't come back, but if it does, don't panic. Make a new plan. Many stage 4 patients are surviving. You can too. Because most immunotherapy trials are for Metastatic Cancer (meaning those with a recurrence), you will now have more options available. Do not jump into more chemo. Explore immunotherapy or perhaps a combination. It can return to your lymph nodes or another site. It can return to an organ also. Do not jump into an APR surgery if it returns to your original site. That may be the first piece of advice given to you. Get a few opinions. They will likely differ dramatically. If you must have surgery, find a way to embrace it. Many survivors are living full and happy lives after colostomies. The surgeries are very advanced and can save your life. There is a survivor's group for those with colostomies that can help.

If feelings of "why me" plague you, then you need to 'give back.' You may question this advice and wonder what gift you have been awarded that requires you to give something back. Unbelievably, my life has more meaning now. I feel like I have been given a gift. It's like a veil has been lifted from over my eyes, and I see things more clearly. I used to go through life wondering what purpose I had. I now understand my purpose. Would this have been possible if not for my illness? All those minor things that used to irritate me are now understood for their trivialities. All those judgments I used to pass onto others are now transformed into empathy. I have truly been given a gift—the gift of clarity.

Tips For Those Newly Diagnosed with Any Cancer

- GET SECOND OPINIONS

- KEEP ODDS IN PERSPECTIVE

- LET YOUR EMOTIONS OUT

- ADDRESS STRESS IMMEDIATELY

- BELIEVE IN THE MIND/BODY CONNECTION

- DETOXIFY

- METABOLICALLY STARVE YOUR CANCER

- CONSIDER _ALL_ OPTIONS INCLUDING CLINICAL TRIALS AND OTHER CANCER CENTERS

- PREPARE YOUR BODY FOR TREATMENT

- DRINK AS MUCH CLEAN, PURE WATER AS POSSIBLE

- OPTIMIZE YOUR IMMUNE SYSTEM

- CHANGE YOUR DIET RADICALLY TO ANTI-CANCER – CONSIDER GREEN/KETO

- GET AN _EXPERIENCED_ TEAM READY

- PROPERLY RESEARCH EVERYTHING IMPORTANT

- WRITE THINGS DOWN – KEEP A JOURNAL

- PRACTISE POSITIVITY AND GRATITUDE

- ADDRESS DEPRESSION IMMEDIATELY

- TAKE AND ASK FOR HELP

- BE YOUR OWN ADVOCATE

- JOIN SUPPORT GROUPS

- KEEP MOVING – EXERCISE OFTEN

- FORGIVE PAST GRIEVANCES

- LOVE YOURSELF

- GIVE BACK

Books I Recommend

The Gift of Cancer by Brenda Michaels

How to Starve Cancer by Jane McLelland

Radical Remission by Kelly Turner

Immune System Booster Affirmations by Stephens Hyang

Cracking Cancer Toolkit by Jeffrey Dach MD

Cancer, A Second Opinion by Dr. Josef Issels

The Breakthrough by Charles Graeber

The Metabolic Approach to Cancer by Nasha Winters

Keto Diet for Cancer by Toma Radu

Cancer is Not a Disease by Andreas Moritz

Never Fear Cancer Again by Raymond Francis, M.Sc.

Chris Beat Cancer by Chris Wark

The Immunotherapy Revolution by Jason R. Williams, MD, DABR

How Not to Die by Michael Greger, MD

The Gerson Therapy by Charlotte Gerson and Morton Walker, DPM

Quick Reference Guide

i https://en.wikipedia.org/wiki/Christine_Blasey_Ford

ii https://en.wikipedia.org/wiki/Dazed_and_Confused_(film)

iii https://budwigcenter.com/the-budwig-diet/

iv https://genius.com/Israel-kamakawiwoole-somewhere-over-the-rainbow-lyrics

v https://www.nccih.nih.gov/health/naturopathy

vi Donald Trump Access Hollywood tape - Wikipedia

vii https://my.clevelandclinic.org/health/diseases/11901-hpv-human-papilloma-virus

viii https://www.webmd.com/women/what-is-leep-procedure

ix https://gerson.org/

x https://www.chrisbeatcancer.com/

xi https://www.analcancerfoundation.org/

xii https://medigence.com/treatment/abdominoperineal-resection#:~:text=Abdominoperinea

xiii https://www.mskcc.org/cancer-care/integrative-medicine/herbs/insulin-potentiation-therapy

xiv Is Chemo Worth It? New Test May Tell (webmd.com)

xv Active Hexose Correlated Compound (AHCC): Overview, Uses, Side Effects, Precautions, Interactions, Dosing and Reviews (webmd.com)

xvi https://en.wikipedia.org/wiki/Nivolumab

xvii https://www.webmd.com/cancer/rick-simpson-oil-for-cancer-overview

xviii https://www.cureyourowncancer.org/corrie-yellands-story-beating-anal-and-skin-cancer-with-cannabis-oil.html

xix https://thesocialmedwork.com/diseases

xx https://clinicaltrials.gov/ct2/show/NCT04287868

xxi https://reboundercanada.com/the-lymphatic-system/

[xxii] https://www.utktechnology.com/2018/08/23/understanding-far-infrared-rays-and-their-benefits-for-cancer/

[xxiii] https://vibralightandwellness.com/photon-genie/

[xxiv] https://my.clevelandclinic.org/health/diagnostics/4952-esophageal-manometry-test

[xxv] https://harmonyintegrativemedicine.com/

[xxvi] https://drjoedispenza.com/

[xxvii] https://en.wikipedia.org/wiki/Psychic_detective

[xxviii] https://herecomesthesun927.com/2016/11/14/dear-every-cancer-patient-i-ever-took-care-of-im-sorry-i-didnt-get-it/

[xxix] https://healthprep.com/featured/everything-you-need-to-know-about-eye-movement-desensitization-and-reprocessing-the-new-type-of-psychotherapy

[xxx] https://clincancerres.aacrjournals.org/content/clincanres/6/1/1.full.pdf

[xxxi] https://www.mskcc.org/cancer-care/diagnosis-treatment/cancer-treatments/radiation-therapy/what-imrt

Made in the USA
Las Vegas, NV
12 November 2021